Ketogenic Diet
for Two

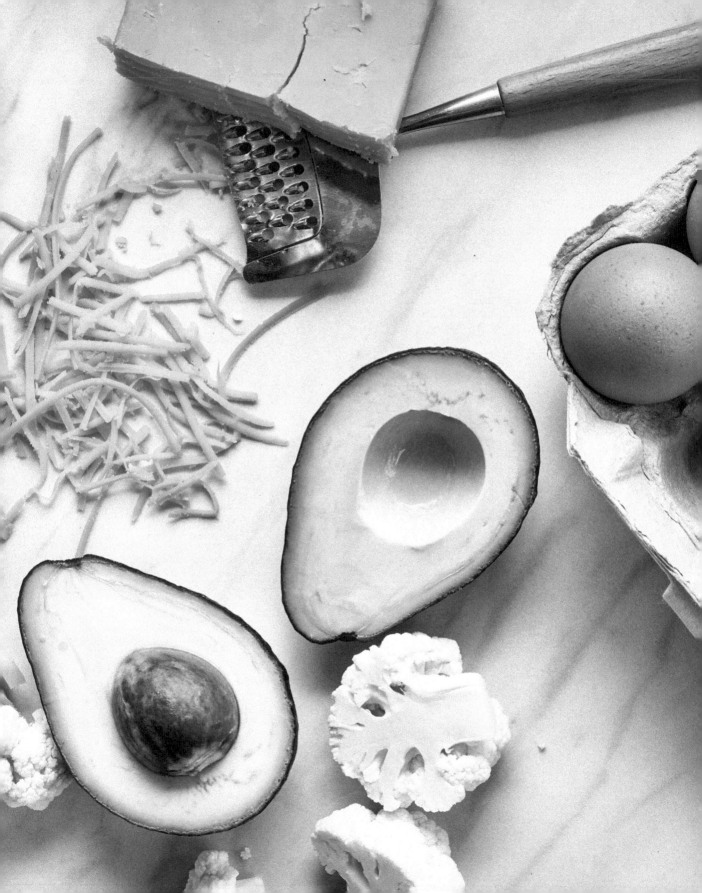

Ketogenic Diet for Two

100 High-Fat, Low-Carb Recipes Portioned for Pairs

THOMAS MARTENS

PHOTOGRAPHY BY ANTONIS ACHILLEOS

ROCKRIDGE
PRESS

To Olivia, without whom
I'd have never learned to cook for two.

Interior and Cover Designer: Carlos Esparza
Art Producer: Meg Baggott
Editor: Anne Lowrey
Production Manager: Holly Haydash
Production Editor: Sigi Nacson

Photography © 2020 Antonis Achilleos
Food styling by Rishon Hanners

ISBN: Print 978-1-64739-176-8 | Ebook 978-1-64739-177-5

R0

Contents

Foreword

When it comes to the keto diet, getting started is always the most frustrating part. More often than not, people are willing to try eating keto, only to give up when the cravings kick in or it starts to feel too repetitive. I myself struggled with similar issues as I began using a ketogenic diet for weight loss. Through Tom's recipes and coaching, I was able to overcome these hurdles that can trip up a diet in an instant.

Tom had started the diet about a year before me and, concerned for my health and well-being, convinced me to try keto. He dove deep into the world of keto, researching the science behind it and discovering how it worked, down to the molecular level. He is always trying to find ways to cook food that will help ease the struggle of dieting. He has become a "black sheep" of keto for going against the standard flow.

On YouTube, he has been helping people by showing them that they don't have to be overly restrictive to get great results; that there are ways to have the food you crave while staying keto. Because of his tips, tricks, and recipes, I've lost over 100 pounds. With the exception of the occasional cheat, I'm still going strong.

His recipes and constant support helped me keep my focus through the cravings and blandness of common recipes. He has made food that looked like it should have been loaded with carbs—the things you crave on keto, like bread, breading, pasta, donuts, chocolate, cakes, and pizza—and turned them keto-friendly. Whenever I would visit, Tom would cook things for me to test out. I became the test subject to his mad scientist, and I'm much better for it.

His are no ordinary recipes. On this diet, you have to be creative. Tom has designed the recipes in this book to show that there are many delicious meals and options in what, at face value, often feels like a restricted way of eating.

—Robert L. Chinn III

Introduction

I wrote this cookbook to help you and a diet partner succeed on a ketogenic diet. Though not everyone comes to keto for the same reasons, my aim is to provide you with the knowledge and recipes necessary to meet the goals that brought you and your diet partner to it.

First, let me tell you a little bit about myself and how I found keto. I am Thomas Martens, the founder of Black Sheep Keto. I research and discuss all things keto through my YouTube videos and website, blacksheepketo.com. Though I'm not a nutritionist or dietitian, I have been researching and experimenting with different forms of ketogenic diets since 2015. My knowledge comes from reading countless research papers, attending presentations from the top researchers in the field, and coaching many people who are starting their keto journeys.

I myself am a keto weight-loss success story. Before I started this diet, I weighed roughly 325 pounds and was starting to see the negative effects of my excess weight on my life. I had tried countless ways to control my weight, but nothing worked over the long term. This all changed when I first heard about keto from a coworker of mine. He had experienced some medical conditions caused by his weight, and his doctor had suggested that he try the ketogenic diet. Like most people, I thought it was absolutely crazy at first. The diet went against everything I had ever been taught about eating. I saw how well it was working for him, though, and it occurred to me that maybe the information I had been listening to about food my whole life was wrong. The more I researched, the more I was convinced that there was something great about the keto diet.

When I first started eating keto, I made every mistake you can think of. This was 2015, and there wasn't much keto information available. For me, the learning curve was steep, but with enough digging through research papers and medical journals I was able to tweak my diet into something sustainable and successful. When my then-girlfriend (now wife) Olivia saw the results I had, she decided to also give it a shot. Eating keto as a couple had its challenges, but it also made accountability much easier. Fast-forward two years: she and I have lost 50 pounds and 125 pounds, respectively. We have both kept the weight off to this day.

After almost five years on keto, we have perfected our method for doing the keto diet for two. Like anything worth doing, it has its challenges. Calculating macros and cooking meals for two people can be harder than it seems. Most recipes create too much food, and always eating leftovers can get boring.

I've combined my experience with and research into solving these problems to create the methods contained in this book. I wish both of you the best of luck as you start your keto journey together. Let's begin.

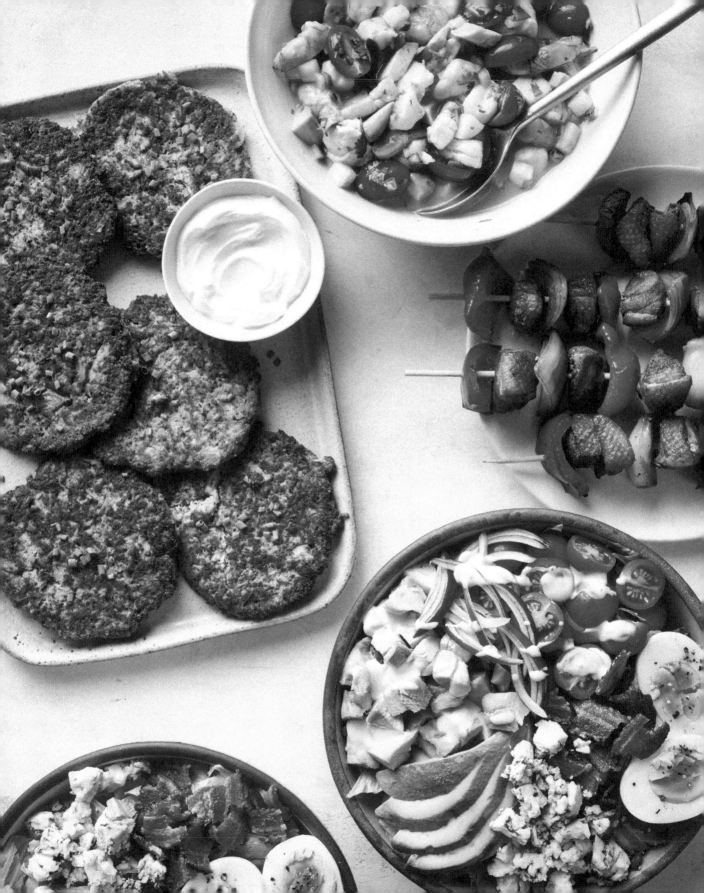

CHAPTER ONE

Why Go Keto?

If you've ever researched keto, you know there are a lot of opinions floating around about how to follow it. This can make starting keto quite overwhelming and intimidating, but it doesn't need to be.

I have boiled down the essential information into a simple, understandable process. We'll also discuss some of the reasons people choose to live a ketogenic lifestyle. Though there are many more reasons than I can mention in this book, some of the ones that we talk about might surprise you.

What Is the Ketogenic Diet?

A ketogenic diet is any diet in which your body is naturally producing ketones for fuel. This is accomplished by limiting your consumption of carbohydrates. But how does it work?

Your body has a defined order in which it utilizes its available energy sources. Carbohydrates are your body's equivalent of rocket fuel—they are essentially the first fuel source that your body looks for. The glucose produced from carbohydrates is very fast burning, which often leads to inconsistent energy levels. Next, your body looks to ketones (produced from fat) for fuel. Ketones, in contrast, are like your body's equivalent of a campfire. They will burn for a long time and produce a consistent supply of energy.

Knowing that your body will burn carbohydrates first probably gives you a good idea of how to get your body to produce ketones: simply *don't* give your body enough carbohydrates to go to them first for fuel. Restricting your carbohydrate intake while increasing your intake of quality fats creates an ideal situation for your liver to start producing ketones, which puts your body into the metabolic state of ketosis.

It would be amazing if there were a magic number of carbohydrates you should consume to stay in ketosis, but every body is different. The good news is: You really don't need to worry about consuming too few carbohydrates, since your body can create glucose as needed through a process known as gluconeogenesis. I'll talk more about that process later in this chapter.

Many people will say that "you can't have X on keto," but based on the definition of a keto diet, combined with the science of how your body reaches ketosis, statements like that are generally wrong. People follow the ketogenic diet for different purposes, including medical reasons, which can carry a different set of restrictions. A lot of information specific to those cases has made its way into the mainstream keto industry. I find that unless you need to avoid specific foods for a medical reason, limiting what you eat generally overcomplicates things and makes the diet harder to stick to. My guidance is to ask yourself: "Is this going to knock me out of ketosis?" If a food has low net carbs and/or a low glycemic index, then it is part of a general keto diet. Otherwise, I would avoid that food.

Low Carb, High Fat

The four words *low carb, high fat* summarize what you need to eat to follow a ketogenic diet. Applying this concept to every meal will make eating keto much easier.

Keeping carbs low guarantees that your body stays in a state of ketosis. Making sure that your fat ratio is high enough gives your body enough available fat to produce ketones. When looking at ingredient labels, this principle is incredibly easy to apply. First, check that the *net carb count* on the product is low. Net carbs are calculated by taking the total carbs and subtracting any fiber or sugar alcohols. Next, verify that the *fat content* is higher than the protein. This ensures that you get a high fat intake while keeping your protein at a moderate level.

Keeping your protein at a moderate level is also important. If you consume an extreme excess of protein, your body can convert this into more glucose than you might want. This is the reason for keeping your fat content higher than the protein. Another simple rule is to stick with dark green vegetables. This will eliminate pretty much all the starchy vegetables and ensure that you get plenty of micronutrients in your diet.

Like me when I first heard about keto, you may have some concerns about the safety of eating a ketogenic diet. One of the first issues that people raise is the potentially increased cholesterol levels that are sometimes associated with eating keto. There are many articles that suggest that modern science doesn't understand the role of cholesterol as much as we think. A study published in the *Journal of the American College of Cardiology* in 2003 showed that individuals with chronic heart failure and a high cholesterol level have a better chance of surviving than those with a lower cholesterol level. As research evolves, it is important to talk to your doctor and follow the recommendations that they make based on your unique situation.

The next concern that I hear quite often is related to getting the right vitamins. This likely comes from that stereotypical belief that people on a keto diet eat slabs of cheese wrapped in bacon, deep-fried, and topped with butter. While that would technically be keto, so is a roasted chicken leg quarter and a side of broccoli. Focus on eating high-vitamin, non-starchy vegetables with your meals.

Macronutrients

Macronutrients—or macros, for short—are essentially the parts of your food that contain calories. The three macros that people commonly track are protein, carbs, and fat. Fat contains 9 calories per gram, while protein and carbs contain only 4. For the sake of completeness, alcohol is a fourth macronutrient, with roughly 7 calories per gram.

A net carb is simply the total carbs minus fiber and certain sugar alcohols, since neither is digested. If you were to read the nutrition label on a product, multiply each macro by its respective caloric value, and add up the results, you would get the total calorie amount. It may be off slightly for commercial products, since they tend to round the numbers. I'll describe more about how to calculate and plan your macros in the next chapter.

The Benefits of Going Keto

The ketogenic diet is often associated with weight loss because of its effectiveness, but that's not the only reason people choose to eat keto. There are numerous medical conditions that the ketogenic diet has been shown to help with. One of the most notable conditions is epilepsy. Studies have been done extensively and show that going on the ketogenic diet greatly reduces or even stops seizures. This is especially great news for the population that suffers with forms of epilepsy that do not respond well to drug treatments.

Another medical condition that has been shown to benefit from a ketogenic diet is diabetes. In fact, there are many accounts of type 2 diabetes being completely reversed using a ketogenic diet. The benefits are also visible in type 1 diabetics through lower blood sugar levels. If you suffer from diabetes, I highly encourage you to talk to your doctor about using a ketogenic diet to help control the condition.

There is also significant research being conducted on treating some diseases and damages to the brain with keto. These include, but are not limited to, autism, traumatic brain injuries, and Alzheimer's disease. Beyond brain injuries, you may see people using keto to treat everything from polycystic ovarian syndrome to cancer. If you're interested in using keto to treat any condition, make sure to talk to your doctor about it first.

Lastly, let's talk about the ketogenic diet for weight loss. This is where the ketogenic diet gained its popularity, and for good reason. Many people who have not succeeded with other diets find that a ketogenic diet allows them to lose weight over the long term. It is important to keep realistic expectations, but I have personally witnessed so many success stories that I firmly believe in the power of keto to defeat stubborn body fat.

Pairing Keto with Intermittent Fasting

Intermittent fasting is a technique that you will often see paired with the keto diet because it can drastically increase the results. Beyond weight loss, other health benefits from fasting include reduced insulin resistance, decreased inflammation, and even improved brain function. Many people use the keto diet for any combination of these reasons, so pairing it with intermittent fasting is a logical choice.

If you're new to fasting, I recommend starting with a 16:8 fast, meaning that you fast for 16 hours per day and eat all your calories within an 8-hour window. This is easiest to accomplish by simply skipping breakfast, but there is no right or wrong time of day to have your eating window. If you become comfortable with a 16:8 fast, then you may even consider a technique known as OMAD, or "one meal a day." This is my personal technique when losing weight, and I absolutely love it. I find that my energy levels are high throughout the day, and I can have a large, satisfying meal even on a calorie-restricted diet.

It is important to stay hydrated while fasting. I'm also a big fan of drinking various zero-calorie electrolyte drink mixes. These electrolytes will keep your energy levels high during your fast. I do not recommend that anyone do a "dry" fast. This is essentially fasting without water, and I do not consider it to be safe. You may see advocates for it on the internet, but I have found no benefits of dry fasting that justify the risk. Speaking of risk, fasting in general isn't for everyone. If you are recovering from an eating disorder, are pregnant or breastfeeding, or are generally malnourished, I would not recommend attempting to fast.

Eating the Keto Way

When you start following a ketogenic diet, there are a few tricks that will make it much easier. The first is focusing on whole foods. There are many products you can find at your local store that are labeled as keto. It's usually noted in huge letters, and there's some algorithm on the back explaining why it is keto. Here's the funny part: a lot of them aren't keto. Some of those products contain ingredients that will knock you out of ketosis. The easiest way to avoid falling into this trap, until you know what to look for, is to avoid packaged foods altogether. Focus on buying whole ingredients and cooking delicious meals with them.

Now that you're looking at the right foods, let's ensure you and your diet partner are drinking enough water. This is a great thing to remind each other of, because it's easy to forget. When you're in a state of ketosis, your body isn't retaining as much water. This is because you have eliminated the glycogen that your body created from consuming carbohydrates. This glycogen binds to water molecules and causes your body to retain it. Since we don't have this glycogen to store excess water, keto dieters often need to increase their regular water consumption.

Electrolytes are singlehandedly the best thing you can ingest to improve your transition to a keto diet. If you've ever heard of the "keto flu," then you've likely seen someone describe an electrolyte shortage. The symptoms are mostly headaches and lethargy, but reports will vary. Fortunately, all this can be avoided by getting enough sodium, potassium, and magnesium in your diet. Some people find that it is easiest to supplement these electrolytes, but you shouldn't need to. Sodium can be obtained through salting your food with a quality sea salt. Potassium and magnesium are available in most dark green vegetables. Try to keep these items in your diet, and you'll be just fine.

We also need to look at the importance of choosing quality ingredients. You can do the ketogenic diet with low-cost, low-nutritional-value ingredients, but there is something to be said about using quality ingredients. A study published in the *Journal of the American College of Nutrition* in 2004 showed that many commercial crops have seen a decrease in nutrient contents since the 1950s. This means that a lot of the micronutrients you would get from vegetables have become less potent in those same vegetables, so choosing quality is important. The same can be said for your meat choices. In the keto community, there is a large debate over grass-fed versus grain-fed beef, but grass-fed does typically contain more vitamin A, vitamin E, and omega-3s. Grass-fed beef often tastes better and has a higher fat content, too. When it comes to the quality of your ingredients, buy the best you can find and afford.

If you're not going to be incorporating fasting into your keto diet, then you might start looking into keto snacks. I would still stress the importance of quality, nutrient-dense foods for your snacks, but they should also be satiating. It's very easy to exceed your daily caloric intake while snacking on food that doesn't make you feel full. For this reason, I recommend snacking on things like eggs, vegetables, meats, and cheeses. These foods score high on the satiety index and will help keep you feeling full.

Feeling full is also a key component of weight loss. If losing weight is one of the goals you have for starting a keto diet, then you should consider incorporating foods that provide a lot of volume in relation to their caloric content. Take, for example, the Cobb salad (I am a huge fan). The lettuce provides a lot of food volume, while the toppings can provide me with the fats and proteins I need to maintain ketosis. Salads aren't the only source of volume, but most of them are going to include many low-calorie, low-carb vegetables.

Foods to Choose

When choosing foods to eat on a keto diet, the most important thing to remember is to keep the fats high and the carbs low. There are far too many foods you can eat on a keto diet for me to list them all, but here are a few categories to get you started.

Meats: All meat can be worked into a ketogenic diet with ease. You should keep an eye on the protein-to-fat ratio, but a high-protein meat can be accompanied with a fatty sauce.

Dark green vegetables: These should make up most of the vegetables you eat because they contain a lot of the micronutrients and electrolytes that your body needs.

Cauliflower: Cauliflower is great to use in place of potatoes. It is healthy, low in carbs, and very versatile.

Eggs: While there are some carbs in eggs, they are minimal. Eggs also contain all amino acids and are quite satiating.

Cheese: Cheese is a great source of fat, and it goes well on almost anything. It's also relatively cheap, for those of us on a budget.

Nut butters: Peanut butter is totally fine in moderation, but you should look at adding other nut butters to your diet that might be slightly lower in carbs. If you've never tried them, give almond butter or coconut butter a try!

Foods to Lose

This is probably the part that you're scared to read. The keto diet has gained a reputation for being incredibly restrictive, but trust me when I say that there is a substitute for almost everything.

Grains: This is probably the hardest one for people to give up, but you need to ditch the bread, pasta, and rice.

Beans: Beans and legumes, including peanuts, can be higher in carbs than you think.

Starchy vegetables: Though there are a ton of vegetables that you can eat on keto, you'll want to avoid the starchy ones, like corn, white potatoes, and sweet potatoes.

Sugar: I recommend familiarizing yourself with the common names for sugar, then avoiding them at all costs. As a rule of thumb, if it rhymes with "gross" (dextrose, fructose, etc.), then it is probably a sugar. This includes the natural sugars that come from fruits.

Soda: It might taste amazing, but it is loaded with sugars. Try swapping it out for a sugar-free carbonated water if you're craving the fizz.

Can We Drink Alcohol on Keto?

Drinking alcohol on keto is doable, but you need to be careful. It's important to limit yourself, and also to wait until you're fully adapted to your keto diet. For most people, the effects of alcohol are much different while on keto than they were before beginning this diet. You will likely not have the tolerance to alcohol you used to have. This can make it much cheaper to go out drinking with your friends, but it's a bit of a surprise if you're not expecting it.

So, what can you drink on keto? As a rule of thumb, stick with unflavored, distilled alcohol mixed with a zero-calorie mixer. Something like a whiskey and diet cola or a vodka and soda water (tonic water contains sugar). If you must have beer, Michelob Ultra and Corona Premier are safe options, with fewer than 3 net carbs per bottle.

Go-to Keto Favorites

Up until this point I've stressed the importance of trying to work with whole ingredients. While this is ideal, a lot of us don't have time to always do that. For this reason, I wanted to provide here a list of the things I believe will save you some time while keeping it keto.

Cauliflower rice: If you've ever tried to make cauliflower rice yourself, you know that it can take a ton of effort. Save yourself the time, and buy it pre-riced in your local freezer section.

Guacamole cups: Avocados are an amazing source of fat and nutrients. Unfortunately, they turn from being too hard to overripe practically instantly. To avoid the wasted ingredients and money, I just buy my avocado in guacamole cups.

Cheese sticks: Buying packaged cheese sticks will save you time and make tracking the macros much easier.

Keto Brick: This is probably my favorite portable keto food. The Keto Brick, a meal replacement bar, is shelf stable, can provide multiple servings, and has fantastic macros. They must be ordered from their website, ketobrick.com, but they're well worth it.

Fat Snax: When you're in need of a keto treat, Fat Snax provides awesome keto cookies that are low in carbs and high in fat. They can be purchased at specialty stores and online at fatsnax.com.

Miracle Noodles: These are a great keto noodle substitute made from the konjac plant and can be found at both Asian grocery stores and supermarkets.

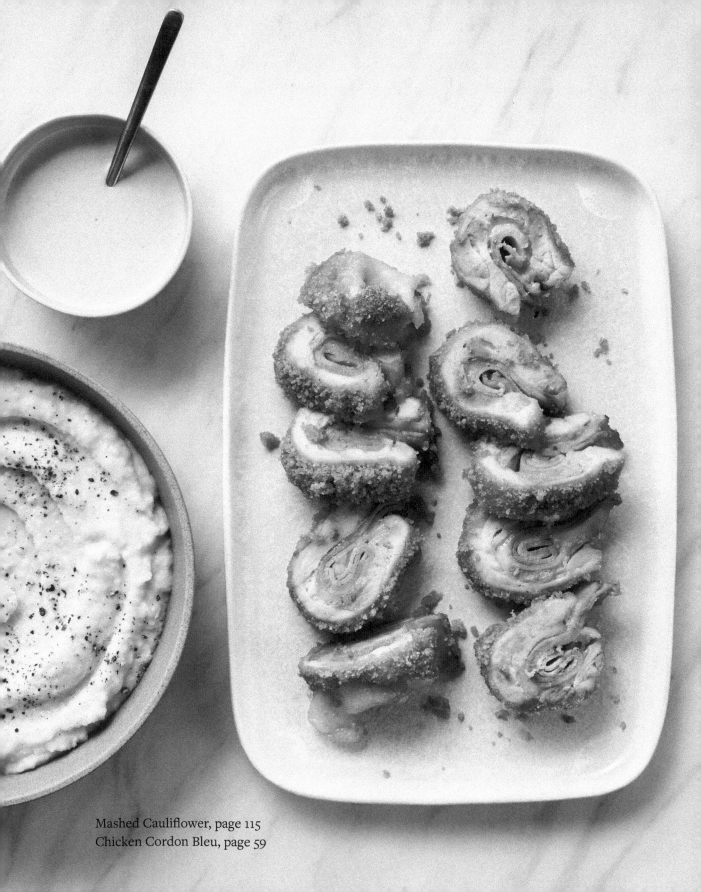

Mashed Cauliflower, page 115
Chicken Cordon Bleu, page 59

CHAPTER TWO

Keto for Two

We'll now dive into the specifics of planning your keto diet. Whether you're starting this journey yourself or beginning it with a partner, I want to provide you with the tools you need to achieve success. In this chapter, I cover everything from figuring out your macros to stocking your pantry. At the end of it, you'll be ready to start cooking and eating keto.

Getting into Ketosis, Together

The support of a diet partner can make the process of getting into ketosis a lot easier. While you're adapting to a ketogenic diet, having that support system is critical to success. I highly encourage you to support each other and, when necessary, call each other's bluff. The initial process of getting into ketosis can take anywhere from three days to a week. It varies a little bit from person to person, but it should be less than a week.

When starting a ketogenic diet, it is important to follow it strictly. This gets you through that transition phase as quickly as possible. A lot is going on inside your body. It's burning through sugar that has been stored. Once that glucose storage is used up, your body will start making ketones! No magic shake that you find on the internet is going to make this process go any faster, despite what some claim. However, a little bit of cardio can speed the process, because you're burning that glucose as fuel. Once you're in ketosis, just keep doing what you're doing, and you'll stay there. This does, however, bring up the question: "How do I know when I'm in ketosis?"

Getting into ketosis for the first time can feel a little bit mysterious. You know the process is taking place inside your body, but you're unable to confirm the results. For this reason, I recommend getting a blood ketone meter. They've come down a lot in cost, making them an affordable way to verify that you're in ketosis. Don't waste your money on urine strips. Simply being hydrated can make the concentration of ketones in your urine low. On the other end of that, if you're dehydrated, the number will go up. I find the blood ketone meter to be much more reliable.

Planning Your Macros

When following a ketogenic diet, eating the proper macronutrient ratio is the key to success. These ratios can change slightly based on individual preference, but I recommend starting with the classic **75 percent fat, 20 percent protein, and 5 percent carbohydrate ratio.** This means that 75 percent of the calories you consume should be coming from a quality fat source, 20 percent from protein, and

5 percent from carbohydrates. Notice that the ratio applies to the *calories* from those sources, not the number of grams.

In order to calculate the grams in each macronutrient you need, we also need to estimate your body's caloric needs. This number can vary greatly from person to person, so make sure that both halves of your "Keto for Two" duo identify their caloric needs independently. Your individual weight, height, muscle mass, activity level, and even biology will affect the number of calories your body needs to function. If you don't know where to start, I recommend calculating your Total Daily Energy Expenditure (TDEE). Simply find a free TDEE calculator online and plug in the information needed for each of you. The resulting number is your caloric need to stay the same weight. If you're following a keto diet for weight loss, then you should reduce that number by 10 to 20 percent. (Note: When you lose weight, you need to recalculate your calories to avoid a "stall.")

This may sound like a lot of math, but thankfully we live in a world where technology has made it all very simple. A food-tracking application for your cell phone will handle it from here. Not only will it calculate your ratio in grams, but it will also always be close by when you need to log a meal. There are many food-tracking apps out there, and they all work roughly the same way. You simply need to find one that allows you to apply custom macros. Once you've done that, supply the app with your desired calories and adjust the macronutrient percentages. Now you're ready to start tracking macros!

It Takes Two to Keto

Starting any new diet or lifestyle can be incredibly difficult. When I first started keto, I was on my own. I had no support, and no one knew what keto was. I can say with 100 percent certainty that having a partner join me on the diet helped dramatically. This was especially the case because we lived together, so we could eliminate all the non-keto temptations from the house. If you have that option, I highly recommend it. You can't eat what isn't there.

When it comes to people other than your diet partner, explaining keto is challenging. To be honest, I don't even tell people I'm on a ketogenic diet. I simply tell them I limit my diet to meats and greens. I have found that this approach never leads to an uncomfortable discussion about keto with people who simply want to tell you not to do it. No one is going to tell you that eating meat and vegetables isn't good for you. Plus, those are really the core foods in a ketogenic diet.

It might not always be easy to talk about your keto journey, but there's one person you should share everything with—your diet partner! That's what they're there for. This is a huge lifestyle change for most people. There is nothing wrong with simply venting. Odds are, both of you are going through the same thing. They might have even found a solution that you can try.

Accountability is probably the biggest benefit in doing the keto diet as two people. It's unrealistic to have someone watching you 24/7 to make sure you're eating the right things. If you're honest with your food-tracking app, then that's just as good. People often try to hide mistakes from their diet partner, but what does that really solve? Share screenshots of your daily macros with each other. You can talk about anything that went wrong and figure out why it happened. The best part about this method is that you don't need to do it in person. Texting your diet partner is also a great option.

Preparing Your Keto Kitchen

Now it's time for the fun part: getting your kitchen keto ready! Whether you live on your own or with your diet partner, I highly recommend getting rid of everything that isn't keto. There are plenty of great food banks that can use your unopened carb-heavy foods. It's best to eliminate the temptations, if you can. If you can't, then I recommend organizing your pantry and refrigerator into keto and "not keto" sections to make your life easier.

Stocking Your Pantry

When it comes to stocking your keto pantry, you simply need to replace the ingredients you already have with keto-friendly varieties. In order to get you started, I'm going to provide you with a list of some things that I like to keep on hand and how they are used on a keto diet.

Olive oil: A great, healthy fat source that provides flavor that complements most dishes. We use this as a general cooking oil.

Basic spices: The key to keeping keto food interesting is to use a wide range of seasonings. A basic spice set should have everything you need to make the recipes in this book.

Pink Himalayan sea salt: Not all salts are equal, and the recipes in this book were created using this type of salt. For best results, get yourself a bag of pink Himalayan sea salt.

Nuts: Did you know that nuts are a great source of fat? Not only do I use them in my cooking, but I also keep a variety of nuts on hand for snacking. For the keto diet, I really like macadamia nuts and almonds, but almost every nut out there is keto friendly.

Shirataki/konjac noodles: These noodles serve as the base for many recipes that would traditionally be cooked with pasta. They also come in a rice shape that I like to keep on hand. Miracle Noodle is a large producer of shirataki noodles, but any brand will work. Look for these in the health food section near the noodle alternatives or in the Asian food section.

Tomato sauce: You can do so much with tomato sauce that I recommend always keeping a can or two on hand. When buying tomato sauce, you really do need to read the ingredients label. Many of them have added sugar hidden in there.

Condiments: I could list a ton of them, but you know what you like. Condiments are a great way to change the flavor of a dish and get you excited to eat it. Just make sure to check the ingredients for any forms of sugar and to verify that the carb count is low.

Almond flour: This is the most common type of flour used in keto recipes. I tend to buy this ingredient in bulk from a big box store in order to save some money. Small bags at specialty stores can be quite expensive.

Xanthan gum: Since the flours used on a ketogenic diet do not have gluten, you need a binding agent to stop baked goods from crumbling to pieces. This is where xanthan gum comes in. It can also be used as a thickening agent instead of ingredients like cornstarch.

Erythritol: Probably the most commonly used sweetener on keto, erythritol is a fantastic item to keep on hand. It can be purchased from most stores and has been well researched.

Stevia: Often, using pure erythritol can lead to a "cooling" aftertaste. The way to avoid that is to use a mixture of stevia and erythritol. It's a small bottle to keep around, and it'll last you forever.

Filling Your Refrigerator

Your refrigerator and freezer doors are going to get a workout on your keto diet. Most of the ingredients used in this book will belong in one of these two places. Here are some ideas of what I keep in my refrigerator and freezer.

Heavy (whipping) cream: Milk has more carbs than you would think. In every case where I would use milk, I substitute heavy cream in a smaller quantity.

Sour cream: Apart from being a delicious topping for a taco, sour cream can be used in baked goods and sauces.

Eggs: Eggs make a great meal on their own and are used quite frequently in keto cooking as a binding agent.

Butter: This is one of my favorite fat sources. I keep a package of butter in both the refrigerator and the freezer so I never run out.

Dark green vegetables: I always try to keep spinach, broccoli, and asparagus on hand. Buying it frozen is a great way to avoid spoilage.

Cauliflower rice: I don't even bother making cauliflower rice anymore because it is so easy to buy it frozen. This can be used to make anything from rice to a substitute for mashed potatoes.

Cheese: Keep your favorite varieties of cheese on hand. I use cheese in many of my recipes to provide some extra fat, but it also makes a fantastic snack.

Ground beef: Stocking up on 80/20 ground beef when it's on sale is a great idea. I like to keep about 1 pound of it in the refrigerator and put my overstock in the freezer. You'll find that ground beef is very versatile and provides excellent keto macros.

Chicken thighs: Chicken thighs are the only cut of chicken you need on keto. They have a higher fat content than other cuts of the bird and can easily be substituted for chicken breast without anyone noticing.

Salmon: With a higher fat content than most other fish, salmon is easily my favorite fish to use on keto.

Keto-Friendly Carb Alternatives

The Standard American Diet, which I like to refer to as SAD, has become incredibly dependent on sweeteners and carbs. They are hidden in absolutely everything, which means that those of us on keto must keep an eye out when choosing foods. As a rule, if the product is thickened or sweetened, then it likely has carbs hidden in it. Therefore, you have to check the label on everything. If the item has a high number of net carbs, then it is best to avoid that food. If you're following a recipe that calls for a carb-filled ingredient, you can sometimes substitute something else with a low net carb count. Here are some common substitutions for you to use everyday cooking.

Ingredient	Amount	Net Carbs	Alternative	Net Carbs
All-purpose flour	1 cup	92 grams	1 cup almond flour + 1 teaspoon xanthan gum	10 grams
All-purpose flour	1 cup	92 grams	⅓ cup coconut flour + ½ teaspoon xanthan gum	6 grams
Granulated sugar	1 teaspoon	4 grams	1 teaspoon erythritol	0 grams
Granulated sugar	½ cup	100 grams	1 teaspoon liquid stevia	0 grams

Ingredient	Amount	Net Carbs	Alternative	Net Carbs
Whole milk	1 cup	12 grams	½ cup heavy (whipping) cream + ½ cup water	4 grams
Potatoes	1 cup	22 grams	1 cup cauliflower	3 grams
Coffee creamer	1 tablespoon	varies	1 tablespoon heavy (whipping) cream + flavored liquid stevia to taste	0.5 gram
Corn syrup	¼ cup	64 grams	2 teaspoons water + ¼ cup allulose. Heat until dissolved.	0 grams
Rice	½ cup	22 grams	½ cup cauliflower rice	1.5 grams
Noodles/ pasta	2 ounces	39 grams	3 ounces shirataki noodles	1 gram

Kitchen Equipment

Throughout the recipes in this book there will be a few pieces of equipment that you need. I'm going to assume you have the generic stuff—pots, pans, knives, cooking utensils, etc. So, in this section, I'm going to focus on inexpensive equipment you might want to purchase for keto cooking specifically. In some cases, these will simply make your life easier; in other cases, it might be necessary to the success of certain recipes. I'll make sure to let you know which ones you absolutely need.

Food processor: This is a must have. It is used extensively to puree ingredients, but it is also great for combining doughs. If there is only one thing you buy, make it a food processor.

Muffin pan: It doesn't need to be anything fancy, but if you don't have one, you should try to get one. I highly recommend silicone muffin pans if you can find them!

Donut pan: This item doesn't get a lot of use, but there is a good reason to have one: keto donuts are a great grab-and-go breakfast. My recipe for them requires a donut pan.

Baking rack: Beyond its purpose of cooling baked goods, if you're cooking something that needs to be crispy on all sides, a baking rack provides an excellent elevated platform for the food to cook on. This item is not necessary, but it is nice to have.

Instant-read thermometer: I'm surprised by the number of kitchens I have been in that do not have a thermometer readily available. This is the best way to guarantee that your food is not over- or undercooked. In the recipes, I provide cook times for all meats, but outside factors can affect the cook time drastically. Having a thermometer will guarantee that you get the best results.

Slow cooker: You can accomplish the same thing with a large pot on the stove, but a slow cooker makes it much easier and requires less supervision. This piece of equipment will mostly be used for making broths and cooking tender meats.

Setting Yourself Up for Success

Success on a ketogenic diet is not something that happens by accident. With some focus and planning ahead, you and your diet partner can work together to achieve your goals.

Meal Planning

When you're just getting started on a keto diet, you probably aren't going to be comfortable enough with keto ingredients to just whip up something on the fly. I find it best to plan my meals for the week in advance. This can be a lot of fun to do with your diet partner. Just take a minute to sit down together and figure out what sounds good. Once you have all the ingredients stocked at home, you can freely decide on what day you want to eat each meal.

Meal prep can also be a very important tool, especially since most people end up eating at least one meal at work. Having premade meals can remove a lot of the temptation to order in food. I like to prepare a large batch of food for the whole week. My wife and I decide on a meal we want for our lunches that week, and then we make a large batch of it together and portion it into bento boxes or storage containers. We then simply grab a box on our way out the door. As a bonus, we know the exact macros that our lunch contains each day, which makes tracking the calories easy.

Dining Out

If you and your diet partner like to go out to eat, then you still can while eating keto. Navigating a restaurant's menu can be a bit tricky at first, but it is totally doable.

The first thing that you should be checking when you consider going out to eat a meal is the nutrition menu. Most chain restaurants have them available on their websites, which means you can go in knowing exactly what you're going to eat. Not only does this remove the temptation of reading the menu while you're there, but you can usually know the exact carb count. However, while the nutrition menu is great for knowing the macros, it doesn't show you the ingredients. Make your best guess to determine what is in the dish, based on the description. When in doubt, ask the server.

If the restaurant doesn't have a nutrition menu, then you need to tread very carefully. Carbs can often be hidden inside unsuspecting dishes. As a rule, I stay away from soups because they are often thickened with flour or cornstarch. I also try to stay away from most sauces, because many of them contain sugar. To keep it safe, I tend to stick to one of these categories when ordering blind:

Salads: I find that most places have a great Cobb salad that requires minimal modifications to make it keto. In most cases, I just ask for no croutons. Cobb salads aren't the only salads that you can have, but they are the most common. Just watch out for sweet fruits, beans, and candied nuts.

Bunless burgers: This is a simple modification that can be made just about anywhere. A burger is usually cheap, and you can physically see the ingredients. Ask for a bun-less or lettuce-wrapped burger to keep it keto. For a side dish, I usually go with green vegetables or a side salad.

Meat and veggies: This is the simplest category for ordering at an unknown restaurant. There is likely some type of meat that is cooked with little or no frills (e.g., steak, grilled chicken, or a pork chop). Getting a nice cut of meat with a side of vegetables is an easy way to keep it keto. If there is a vegetable mix, make sure to ask what is in it.

Handling Cravings and Crashes

Everyone falls off the food wagon from time to time. It's nothing to feel ashamed about or embarrassed by. It is a perfectly normal thing that happens on the keto diet. Sometimes this happens because you've been strict with yourself for a while and decide to have a day where you treat yourself to the foods you are missing. Sometimes it's an unexpected situation or it's outside your control. The important thing is to recover from the deviation and minimize the damage.

The first thing we need to talk about is cheat days—or "treat days," as I like to call them. If you're doing keto for weight loss, then sometimes it is okay to have a planned treat. It can be great for your sanity. This, however, can also be a slippery slope for some people. If you're going to do a treat day, it should be a very rare occurrence limited to one meal. I've found that the amount of carbs that I might get from a single treat meal is usually not enough to stop ketosis altogether. However, when you have multiple treat meals over multiple days you might get completely knocked out of ketosis.

Aside from planned times when you're not following your diet, occasionally temptation might get the best of you. It has happened to me more times than I can count. I encourage you to accept that it has happened, and try to figure out how to prevent it in the future. Sometimes prevention is as simple as finding a substitute for a food that you crave. If you're having trouble finding a solution, though, ask your diet partner! Between the two of you, I'm sure a solution can be found.

Keto Meals for Two, Made Simpler

My goal with the recipes in this book is to make cooking keto for two much simpler. Traditional recipes aren't designed for just two people, which means there is the temptation to overeat or you have lots of leftovers. The recipes in this book are designed to provide only two to four portions of a dish, while keeping the macros on track for a keto diet. Make sure to double-check the portions to guarantee that you're getting the proper macros.

If you and your partner have very different caloric needs, then some of the recipes serving three or four can help fill that gap in calories. The net carb counts for each of these recipes are low enough that you should have no problem staying under your limit as you combine them to create your meals for the day. Additionally, the macros for each recipe have been accurately calculated, taking a lot of the guesswork out of cooking. If you follow these recipes and track everything, then you should have no problem cooking a keto diet for two people.

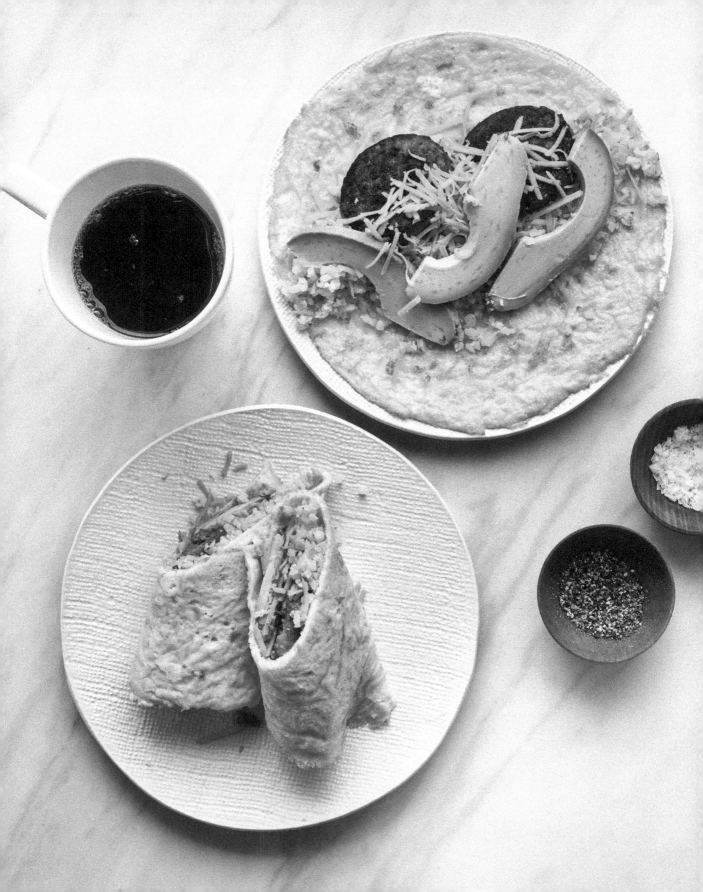

CHAPTER THREE

Breakfast and Eggs

Berry Breakfast Parfaits

EGG FREE, UNDER 30 MINUTES, VEGETARIAN

Serves 2
Prep Time: 5 minutes

½ cup mixed blueberries,
raspberries, sliced
strawberries, and/or
blackberries, fresh or
frozen (and thawed)
1 cup Two Good
vanilla yogurt
½ cup walnut halves
or pieces

If you're looking for a simple and fresh keto breakfast option, look no further. These mixed berry parfaits are quick to make, totally customizable, and most importantly, delicious. Don't feel restricted by the recipe that I have written here. You can also your favorite nuts, berries, or flavor of yogurt to make this your own.

1. In 2 small glass jars or bowls, place a layer of mixed berries.

2. Top this layer with a small amount of yogurt, followed by a layer of nuts.

3. Continue to alternate layers until all the ingredients are evenly distributed between the 2 portions.

Ingredient Tip: Most yogurts are not keto. I have found the Two Good brand is a great keto yogurt option that is available in most places. You can also look for Kite Hill plain unsweetened almond yogurt, but only the plain flavor is keto-friendly.

Macronutrients: 66% Fat, 12% Protein, 21% Carbs

Per serving: Calories: 259; Total Fat: 20g; Protein: 8g; Total Carbohydrates: 14g; Fiber: 3g; Erythritol: 0g; Net Carbs: 11g

Scrambled Egg Cups

NUT FREE, UNDER 30 MINUTES

Serves 4
Prep Time: 10 minutes
Cook Time: 18 minutes

Coconut oil cooking spray
4 large eggs
1 tablespoon heavy
   (whipping) cream
Pink Himalayan sea salt
Freshly ground
   black pepper
¼ cup sliced fresh
   mushrooms
¼ cup chopped
   fresh spinach
2 bacon slices, cooked until
   crisp and crumbled
2 tablespoons
   chopped onion
¼ cup shredded
   cheddar cheese

This recipe was created as my quick-breakfast meal prep. When I inevitably woke up late, I could still have a hot breakfast ready to eat in seconds. An egg cup is essentially an omelet in muffin form. These are loaded with all your favorite breakfast flavors and can be eaten with one hand as you're running out the door, or made fresh any morning.

1. Preheat the oven to 350°F. Spray 4 cups of a muffin pan with the cooking spray.

2. In a medium bowl, whisk the eggs and cream, then season with salt and pepper.

3. In another medium bowl, mix the mushrooms, spinach, bacon, and onion.

4. Spoon the egg mixture evenly into the 4 muffin cups.

5. Top each with some of the bacon mixture. Finally, top the cups with an even sprinkling of cheddar cheese.

6. Bake for 16 to 18 minutes, until the eggs are set.

Storage Tip: Egg cups reheat surprisingly well. Store them in an airtight container in the refrigerator for up to 3 days, then reheat in the microwave when you're ready to eat them.

Macronutrients: 68% Fat, 29% Protein, 3% Carbs

Per serving (1 egg muffin): Calories: 146; Total Fat: 11g; Protein: 10g; Total Carbohydrates: 1g; Fiber: 0g; Erythritol: 0g; Net Carbs: 1g

Ham and Cheese Quiche

Serves 4
Prep Time: 10 minutes
Cook Time: 45 minutes

The key to a great quiche is the crust, and unfortunately that's typically left off of keto quiches. This recipe for our ham and cheese quiche isn't just cheesy, fluffy, and delicious; it also has a crust! With this recipe, you'll never feel like something is missing from a keto quiche again.

For the crust

1½ cups almond flour

5 tablespoons butter, melted

2 teaspoons heavy (whipping) cream

1 teaspoon psyllium husk powder

For the filling

6 large eggs

½ cup heavy (whipping) cream

1 teaspoon pink Himalayan sea salt

½ teaspoon freshly ground black pepper

6 ounces boneless ham, cooked and cubed

1½ cups shredded cheddar cheese, divided

¼ cup chopped onion

1. Preheat the oven to 350°F.

2. **To make the crust:** In a medium bowl, combine the almond flour, butter, cream, and psyllium husk powder. Mix with a fork.

3. In a 9-inch pie dish, form a crust by pushing the crust mixture against the bottom and up the sides of the dish, using the fork. It should be as even in thickness as possible.

4. **To make the filling:** In a medium bowl, whisk together the eggs, cream, salt, and pepper.

5. Stir in the ham, ¾ cup of cheese, and the onion.

6. Pour this mixture into the pie dish.

7. Top with the remaining ¾ cup of cheese.

8. Bake for 40 to 45 minutes, until the center is set. Let rest for 10 minutes, cut into 4 slices, and serve.

Variation Tip: The cubed ham can be substituted with cooked breakfast sausage, crumbled bacon, or even cooked chicken. The cheese can also be substituted with your favorite flavor.

Macronutrients: 76% Fat, 18% Protein, 6% Carbs

Per serving: Calories: 796; Total Fat: 69g; Protein: 35g; Total Carbohydrates: 12g; Fiber: 5g; Erythritol: 0g; Net Carbs: 7g

French "Toast"

NUT FREE, VEGETARIAN

Serves 2
Prep Time: 5 minutes
Cook Time: 25 minutes

4 large eggs, at room
temperature
4 ounces full-fat cream
cheese, at room
temperature
3 tablespoons butter, at
room temperature
¼ teaspoon ground
cinnamon
Keto syrup of choice
(see Tip)

This keto substitute for French toast is a simple mixture of cream cheese, butter, and eggs baked to form soft, bread-like slices that are then toasted on the stovetop. When both sides of the slices are crisped and you've covered them with keto-friendly syrup, you'll have no problem seeing why we call this keto French "toast."

1. Preheat the oven to 350°F.
2. In a food processor or blender, process the eggs, cream cheese, butter, and cinnamon into a smooth batter. Pour the batter into an 8-inch square non-stick baking dish.
3. Bake for 15 to 20 minutes, until a knife inserted into the middle comes out clean.
4. Allow the baked "bread" to cool for about 10 minutes, then cut into 4 equal pieces.
5. Heat a medium nonstick sauté pan or skillet over medium heat. Place the slices in the pan and toast each side for 1 to 2 minutes, until lightly browned. Serve 2 slices on each plate, and top with keto syrup.

Ingredient Tip: I recommend serving this with a keto-friendly maple-flavored syrup. For this, I typically use Walden Farms pancake syrup because it is keto and has zero calories.

Macronutrients: 83% Fat, 14% Protein, 3% Carbs

Per serving: Calories: 490; Total Fat: 46g; Protein: 16g; Total Carbohydrates: 3g; Fiber: 0g; Erythritol: 0g; Net Carbs: 3g

Jelly-Filled Breakfast Strudels

VEGETARIAN

Serves 2
Prep Time: 10 minutes
Cook Time: 25 minutes

For the pastry

¾ cup shredded
  low-moisture
  mozzarella cheese
2 ounces full-fat cream
  cheese, at room
  temperature
1 cup almond flour
1 large egg
4 tablespoons
  stevia-sweetened jelly
  (see Tip)

This recipe for small breakfast strudels has the perfect amount of jelly stuffed into a version of Fathead dough. The Fathead dough, a keto favorite, combines cheese and almond flour to create a chewy, bread-like dough that can hold a sweet filling for an awesome breakfast pastry. Top these with cream cheese frosting to complete the dish.

1. Preheat the oven to 325°F. Have a silicone-lined baking sheet nearby.

2. **To make the dough:** In a large, microwave-safe bowl, combine the mozzarella and cream cheese.

3. Microwave for 1 minute, until the cheese is melted. Then stir to combine.

4. Add the almond flour and egg to the melted cheese. Combine using a rubber scraper, working quickly so the cheese does not cool and harden. (If it starts to harden, reheat in the microwave for 20 seconds, being careful not to cook the egg.)

5. Roll out the dough between 2 pieces of parchment paper to a large rectangle that is between ¼ and ⅛ inch thick.

6. Make 3 even cuts widthwise to form 4 long rectangles of dough.

7. Place 1 tablespoon of jelly in the top half of each rectangle, leaving a little room on the sides.

8. Puncture the non-jellied bottom of each rectangle with a fork. Then, fold this bottom half over the top jellied half.

For the frosting

¼ cup powdered erythritol

2 ounces full-fat cream
cheese, at room
temperature

1 tablespoon butter, at
room temperature

2 teaspoons heavy
(whipping) cream

¼ teaspoon vanilla extract

9. Seal the edges all the way around the square by pressing down with a fork. Transfer the squares to the baking sheet.

10. Bake for 20 to 25 minutes, until the pastry is golden brown.

11. Remove from the oven, and allow to cool for 10 minutes.

12. **To make the frosting:** In a small bowl, combine the erythritol, cream cheese, butter, cream, and vanilla and mix until smooth.

13. With a knife or the back of a spoon, coat the strudels with frosting and enjoy.

Variation Tip: If you can't find stevia-sweetened jelly at your local grocery store, try stuffing the pastries with keto-friendly chocolate chips. If you aren't going to make the frosting, add some sweetener to the dough; the frosting is used to sweeten the whole dish.

Storage Tip: You can freeze any remaining pastries. When you're ready to eat them, simply heat them in a toaster oven.

Macronutrients: 76% Fat, 15% Protein, 9% Carbs

Per serving: Calories: 702; Total Fat: 61g; Protein: 27g; Total Carbohydrates: 16g; Fiber: 6g; Erythritol: 24g; Net Carbs: 10g

Inside-Out Breakfast Burrito

UNDER 30 MINUTES

Serves 2
Prep Time: 10 minutes
Cook Time: 5 minutes

For the wrap

¼ cup shredded
low-moisture
mozzarella cheese
2 large eggs
1 teaspoon coconut flour
Pink Himalayan sea salt
Freshly ground
black pepper
2 teaspoons extra-virgin
olive oil, divided

For the burrito

½ cup cauliflower
rice, cooked
4 ounces breakfast
sausage, cooked
½ cup shredded
cheddar cheese
1 medium avocado, sliced

When I first started a keto diet, I often made breakfast burritos using low-carb tortillas. I soon found a better way—this inside-out breakfast burrito. The "tortilla" is made from the eggs that would normally be inside the burrito and filled with cauliflower rice, sausage, cheese, and avocado. Each bite is guaranteed to be full of flavor.

1. **To make the wrap:** In a medium bowl, whisk together the mozzarella, eggs, and coconut flour. Season with salt and pepper.

2. In an 8-inch skillet, heat 1 teaspoon of olive oil over medium-low heat.

3. Pour half the egg mixture into the pan and rotate the pan to spread it evenly on the skillet bottom.

4. Cook for about 1 minute on each side, flipping once.

5. Remove the egg wrap from the heat and cool.

6. Repeat steps 2 to 5 for the second wrap.

7. **To make the burrito:** Onto each wrap, evenly spread half the cauliflower rice, sausage, cheddar cheese, and avocado.

8. Fold the sides in, roll up like a burrito, and enjoy!

Variation Tip: If you like spicy foods, try this recipe with habanero pepper jack cheese or top the filling with spicy salsa before rolling it up.

Macronutrients: 74% Fat, 18% Protein, 8% Carbs

Per serving: Calories: 654; Total Fat: 55g; Protein: 29g; Total Carbohydrates: 15g; Fiber: 9g; Erythritol: 0g; Net Carbs: 6g

No Oat–Meal

EGG FREE, NUT FREE, UNDER 30 MINUTES, VEGETARIAN

Serves 2
Prep Time: 5 minutes
Cook Time: 5 minutes

2 cups water

¼ cup ground flaxseed

¼ cup protein powder,
   any flavor

2 tablespoons chia seeds

Pinch of pink Himalayan
   sea salt

2 tablespoons butter

2 tablespoons heavy
   (whipping) cream

1 tablespoon granulated
   erythritol

A keto breakfast can be so much more than just eggs and bacon. This keto oatmeal substitute will bring your favorite childhood breakfast into your new way of eating. The flavor and texture are similar to classic oatmeal, but since oats aren't keto, here's a version using keto-friendly ingredients. This recipe gives you the freedom to make it taste like your favorite flavor of oatmeal, so it's sure to end up in your regular rotation.

1. In a medium saucepan, bring the water to a gentle boil.

2. Using a whisk, stir in the flaxseed, protein powder, chia seeds, and salt.

3. Continue to simmer and stir until the mixture reaches the consistency of pudding.

4. Add the butter, cream, and erythritol.

5. Stir until the butter is melted.

6. Remove the saucepan from the heat, and split the cereal between 2 bowls.

7. Add any desired toppings and enjoy!

Variation Tip: You can easily change the flavor profile of this cereal by adding some mix-ins. I recommend nut butter, a keto-friendly maple-flavored syrup, or anything else that sounds delicious to you.

Macronutrients: 76% Fat, 20% Protein, 4% Carbs

Per serving: Calories: 330; Total Fat: 25g; Protein: 15g; Total Carbohydrates: 10g; Fiber: 7g; Erythritol: 6g; Net Carbs: 3g

Blueberry Muffins

VEGETARIAN

Serves 4
Prep Time: 5 minutes
Cook Time: 25 minutes

¾ cup almond flour

3 tablespoons granulated
   erythritol

1 tablespoon ground
   flaxseed

1 teaspoon baking powder

¼ teaspoon pink Himalayan
   sea salt

2 large eggs

3 tablespoons
   butter, melted

⅓ cup fresh or frozen
   blueberries

Muffins are something I never thought I would miss when I started keto. As it turns out, I did miss them—so I created this recipe. The muffins are light and fluffy, but they can still hold a topping of melted butter. The sweetness of the blueberries stands out from the buttery bread, resulting in an amazing homemade blueberry muffin.

1. Preheat the oven to 350°F. Line 4 cups of a muffin pan with paper cupcake liners.

2. In a large bowl, combine the almond flour, erythritol, flaxseed, baking powder, and salt.

3. In a medium bowl, whisk the eggs until lightly beaten. Add the butter and whisk to combine.

4. Pour the wet ingredients into the dry, then mix well to form the batter. Fold in the blueberries.

5. Divide the batter among the 4 lined muffin cups.

6. Bake for about 25 minutes, until the tops are lightly browned.

Variation Tip: This recipe works as a great base for almost any type of muffin. Replace the blueberries with chopped strawberries or keto chocolate chips to make an entirely new meal.

Macronutrients: 77% Fat, 12% Protein, 11% Carbs

Per serving: Calories: 233; Total Fat: 21g; Protein: 7g; Total Carbohydrates: 7g; Fiber: 3g; Erythritol: 9g; Net Carbs: 4g

Egg-Stuffed Avocados

DAIRY FREE, NUT FREE

Serves 2
Prep Time: 5 minutes
Cook Time: 35 minutes

1 large avocado, halved
   and pitted
2 small eggs
Pink Himalayan sea salt
Freshly ground
   black pepper
1 bacon slice, cooked until
   crispy and crumbled

Avocado toast might be a huge craze right now, but everyone's missing out on something even better! This egg-stuffed avocado captures all the flavor of a breakfast avocado toast, with none of the carbs. In addition to looking and tasting great, the dish is loaded with the electrolytes you need on a keto diet.

1. Preheat the oven to 375°F.
2. Using a small spoon, enlarge the hole of the avocado left by the pit so it is roughly 2 inches in diameter.
3. Place the avocado halves cut-side up on a baking sheet.
4. Crack an egg into the well of each half. Season with salt and pepper.
5. Bake for 30 to 35 minutes, until the yolk reaches your preferred texture, 30 minutes for soft and 35 minutes for hard.
6. Sprinkle the bacon crumbles on top and enjoy!

Ingredient Tip: Hall avocados work best here, since they are larger than Hass, but any large avocado will do.

Macronutrients: 68% Fat, 15% Protein, 18% Carbs

Per serving: Calories: 264; Total Fat: 21g; Protein: 10g; Total Carbohydrates: 12g; Fiber: 9g; Erythritol: 0g; Net Carbs: 3g

Glazed Chocolate Donuts

VEGETARIAN

Serves 3
Prep Time: 10 minutes
Cook Time: 20 minutes

For the donuts

Coconut oil cooking spray

½ cup almond flour

¼ cup granulated erythritol

2 tablespoons unsweetened
cocoa powder

¾ teaspoon baking powder

¼ teaspoon xanthan gum

⅛ teaspoon pink Himalayan
sea salt

1 large egg

3 tablespoons heavy
(whipping) cream

2 tablespoons
butter, melted

¼ teaspoon vanilla extract

Just because you're following a ketogenic diet doesn't mean you have to miss out on breakfast treats. These keto chocolate donuts have a similar texture to a cake donut and are similarly topped with a sweet glaze. This recipe will satisfy your morning sweet tooth while keeping you in a state of ketosis.

1. Preheat the oven to 325°F. Spray 3 molds of a donut pan with cooking spray.

2. **To make the donuts:** In a large bowl, combine the almond flour, erythritol, cocoa powder, baking powder, xanthan gum, and salt. Using a whisk, mix well; there should be no clumps.

3. In a small bowl, whisk the egg, cream, melted butter, and vanilla.

4. Pour the wet ingredients into the dry. Whisk until well combined.

5. Portion the dough evenly into these 3 molds.

6. Smooth the donut tops with a wet spoon.

7. Bake for 18 to 20 minutes, until a toothpick inserted in the center comes out clean.

8. Carefully flip the donut pan onto a cooling rack to release the donuts.

9. Let the donuts cool completely before glazing.

For the glaze

2 tablespoons powdered
  erythritol

2 tablespoons
  butter, melted

2 teaspoons heavy
  (whipping)
  cream, warmed

10. **To make the glaze:** In a small bowl, combine the erythritol, butter, and cream and whisk until smooth.

11. Using a spoon or brush, coat each donut with the glaze mixture, then return it to the cooling rack. If you have enough glaze, double-coat them.

12. Let cool for 30 to 60 minutes. The glaze should be firm to the touch, but you can eat the donuts before the glaze dries, if you can't wait.

Variation Tip: A chocolate glaze can be easily made by adding a little cocoa powder to the glaze mixture. Start with 1 teaspoon cocoa and then adjust to your desired chocolate intensity.

Macronutrients: 86% Fat, 7% Protein, 7% Carbs

Per serving: Calories: 331; Total Fat: 33g; Protein: 7g; Total Carbohydrates: 7g; Fiber: 3g; Erythritol: 24g; Net Carbs: 4g

Mixed Berry Smoothie

EGG FREE, NUT FREE, UNDER 30 MINUTES, VEGETARIAN

Serves 2
Prep Time: 5 minutes

½ cup fresh or frozen
  strawberries
½ cup fresh or frozen
  blueberries
½ cup fresh or frozen
  raspberries
1 cup ice cubes
½ cup heavy
  (whipping) cream
½ cup Two Good
  vanilla yogurt
2 tablespoons MCT oil
¼ to ½ cup water,
  as needed

This keto smoothie captures the taste, texture, and bright colors of a traditional smoothie, but keeps the carbs low. To achieve a great fat ratio, the berries are blended into a mixture of cream, yogurt, and MCT oil. With the mixed berry flavor alongside the fats that you need to maintain ketosis, this smoothie is bound to become a favorite.

1. Fill a high-speed blender with the berries, ice cubes, cream, yogurt, and MCT oil.

2. Blend until smooth. If your blender struggles with the thickness, slowly add the water until it begins to blend.

3. Divide the mixture between 2 glasses and enjoy!

Ingredient Tip: Most yogurts are not keto, but Two Good yogurt is a great keto option that is available in many places. Kite Hill plain unsweetened almond yogurt is also keto and widely available.

Macronutrients: 81% Fat, 4% Protein, 15% Carbs

Per serving: Calories: 408; Total Fat: 38g; Protein: 4g; Total Carbohydrates: 16g; Fiber: 4g; Erythritol: 0g; Net Carbs: 12g

Blended Iced Coffee

EGG FREE, NUT FREE, UNDER 30 MINUTES, VEGETARIAN

Serves 2
Prep Time: 5 minutes

2 cups brewed
  coffee, chilled
2 cups ice cubes
½ cup heavy
  (whipping) cream
½ cup canned
  coconut cream
½ teaspoon vanilla extract
¼ teaspoon liquid stevia

If you're a coffee lover like me, then you're in luck with this caffeinated treat. Instead of heading to your corner coffee shop for a blended iced coffee that is most likely loaded with sugar, try making this at home. The ingredients are simple and completely keto, and it's the perfect consistency, with moderate coffee flavor.

Fill a high-speed blender with the coffee, ice cubes, cream, coconut cream, vanilla, and stevia. Blend until smooth. Divide the mixture between 2 glasses and enjoy!

Ingredient Tip: If you cannot find canned coconut cream, you can skim some cream off the top of a can of coconut milk (do not shake before opening the can).

Variation Tip: You can flavor the coffee using various extracts and flavorings. Just ensure that they are sugar-free.

Macronutrients: 91% Fat, 3% Protein, 6% Carbs

Per serving: Calories: 406; Total Fat: 43g; Protein: 3g; Total Carbohydrates: 6g; Fiber: 1g; Erythritol: 1g; Net Carbs: 5g

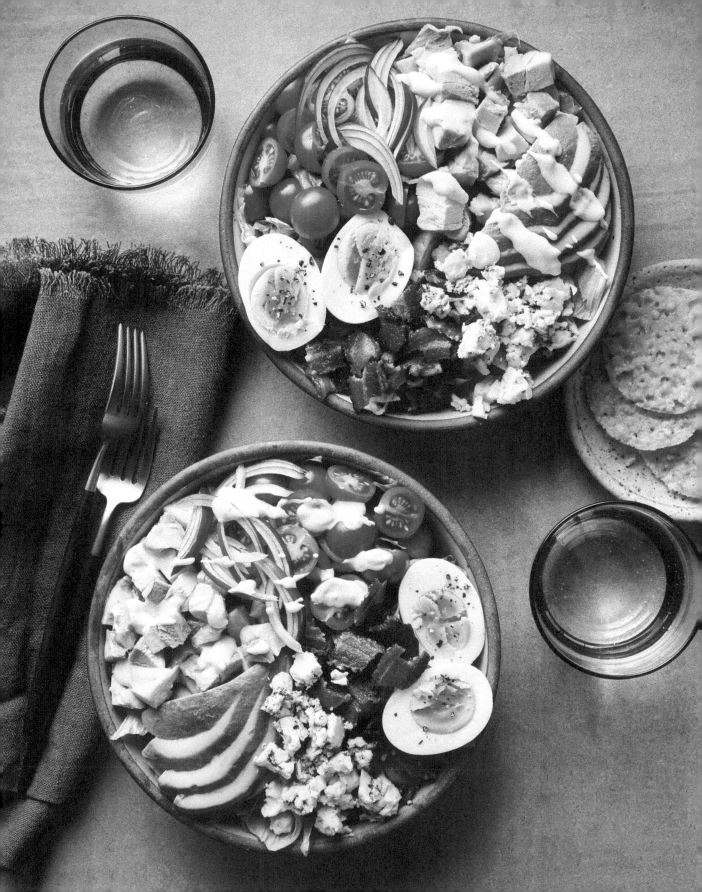

CHAPTER FOUR

Salads and Soups

Caprese Salad

NUT FREE, UNDER 30 MINUTES, VEGETARIAN

Serves 2
Prep Time: 10 minutes

¾ cup cherry tomatoes

4 ounces fresh
mozzarella pearls

2 tablespoons extra-virgin
olive oil

5 to 6 fresh basil leaves

Pink Himalayan sea salt

Freshly ground
black pepper

A caprese salad is probably the easiest salad you're ever going to make. This is simply a mix of fresh mozzarella, tomatoes, basil, olive oil, and pepper. Once combined, these powerful flavors blend to create an amazing salad that is truly greater than the sum of its parts.

1. In a large bowl, toss to combine the tomatoes, mozzarella, and olive oil.

2. Stack the basil leaves, roll them into a cylinder, and then cut into ribbons (chiffonade). Add the basil to the bowl.

3. Toss the ingredients until everything is coated in the dressing. Season with salt and pepper.

Ingredient Tip: Try to get the freshest ingredients you can. Look for bright red and juicy tomatoes when in season. The quality of ingredients can make or break a caprese salad.

Macronutrients: 77% Fat, 18% Protein, 5% Carbs

Per serving: Calories: 300; Total Fat: 26g; Protein: 13g; Total Carbohydrates: 3g; Fiber: 1g; Erythritol: 0g; Net Carbs: 2g

Cobb Salad

NUT FREE, UNDER 30 MINUTES

Serves 2
Prep Time: 10 minutes

½ head romaine
lettuce, chopped

8 ounces boneless, skinless
chicken thighs, cooked
and cubed

2 large eggs, hard-boiled,
peeled, and sliced

⅓ cup cherry
tomatoes, halved

1 avocado, sliced

2 bacon slices, cooked until
crisp and crumbled

¼ medium red onion, sliced
into strips

½ cup blue cheese
crumbles

1 ounce Parmesan crisps

½ cup ranch or blue cheese
dressing

Cobb salad is probably my favorite type of salad for keto. It provides a wide range of flavors to keep your taste buds entertained. From the creamy richness of the avocado to the salty crunch of the Parmesan crisps, this Cobb salad has it all. Even though most Cobb salads are keto, this recipe is designed to give you an extra boost of fat.

1. Fill a large bowl with the romaine lettuce.
2. Top with the chicken, egg, tomatoes, avocado, bacon, red onion, blue cheese crumbles, and Parmesan crisps.
3. Drizzle the dressing on top, and toss well.

Ingredient Tip: Many of the ingredients in the recipe can be bought pre-cut or already cooked. This can save a lot of time when making a Cobb salad.

Macronutrients: 73% Fat, 18% Protein, 9% Carbs

Per serving: Calories: 1070; Total Fat: 88g; Protein: 47g; Total Carbohydrates: 26g; Fiber: 13g; Erythritol: 0g; Net Carbs: 13g

Egg Salad

DAIRY FREE, NUT FREE, UNDER 30 MINUTES, VEGETARIAN

Serves 2

Prep Time: 5 minutes

3 tablespoons mayonnaise

2 teaspoons
  yellow mustard

½ teaspoon dried dill

Pink Himalayan sea salt

Freshly ground
  black pepper

4 large eggs, hard-boiled,
  peeled, and cut into
  ½-inch pieces

1 tablespoon chopped
  fresh chives

Whether you eat it with a spoon or wrap it in a keto tortilla, egg salad makes a fantastic keto meal, and this salad is a beautiful dish that tastes as great as it looks. The dressing is a simple mix of mayonnaise and mustard, but the flavor of dill really brings this dish together.

1. In a medium bowl, combine the mayonnaise, mustard, dill, and salt and pepper to taste.

2. Add in the eggs and chives. Mix until the eggs are coated with the dressing, then serve.

Variation Tip: If you go the tortilla route for enjoying this egg salad, try it topped with a sprinkle of cheddar cheese.

Macronutrients: 79% Fat, 19% Protein, 2% Carbs

Per serving: Calories: 289; Total Fat: 25g; Protein: 13g; Total Carbohydrates: 2g; Fiber: 0g; Erythritol: 0g; Net Carbs: 2g

Beef Taco Salad

EGG FREE, NUT FREE, UNDER 30 MINUTES

Serves 2
Prep Time: 10 minutes
Cook Time: 10 minutes

1 pound ground
  beef (80/20)
1 teaspoon chili powder
½ teaspoon ground cumin
½ teaspoon pink Himalayan
  sea salt
½ teaspoon freshly ground
  black pepper
¼ teaspoon garlic powder
¼ teaspoon onion powder
¼ teaspoon dried oregano
¼ teaspoon paprika
Pinch of cayenne pepper
½ romaine lettuce,
  chopped
1 avocado, sliced
½ cup shredded
  cheddar cheese
½ cup cherry tomatoes,
  halved
1 ounce Parmesan crisps,
  crumbled
¼ cup sour cream
2 teaspoons hot sauce
  of choice

This salad is a go-to in my house. It can be ready in just minutes with ingredients that are always on hand. The slightly spicy blend of flavors is cooled down with a sour cream sauce. It's a great taco salad that has a flavorful and spicy crunch in each bite.

1. In a medium sauté pan or skillet, cook the beef over medium-high heat for 7 to 10 minutes, until browned.

2. Season the meat with the chili powder, cumin, salt, pepper, garlic powder, onion powder, oregano, paprika, and cayenne. Stir until the spices combine with the drippings to coat the meat.

3. Assemble the salad by forming a base of lettuce on 2 plates, then top each with beef, avocado, cheese, tomatoes, and Parmesan crisps (these are like tortilla chips!).

4. In a small bowl, combine the sour cream and hot sauce. Drizzle the dressing over the salads and serve.

Variation Tip: Guacamole is a great substitute for fresh avocado, and the store-bought version makes this salad easier. Just take a look at the ingredients listed on the container to make sure that it is keto.

Macronutrients: 73% Fat, 24% Protein, 3% Carbs

Per serving: Calories: 968; Total Fat: 47g; Protein: 56g; Total Carbohydrates: 17g; Fiber 9g; Erythritol: 0g; Net Carbs 8g

Burger in a Bowl

EGG FREE, NUT FREE, UNDER 30 MINUTES

Serves 2
Prep Time: 10 minutes
Cook Time: 10 minutes

1 pound ground
 beef (80/20)
¼ teaspoon pink Himalayan
 sea salt
¼ teaspoon freshly ground
 black pepper
¼ cup mayonnaise
2 tablespoons
 sugar-free ketchup
2 tablespoons
 yellow mustard
1 tablespoon dill relish
1 (8-ounce) bag
 shredded lettuce
½ cup sliced red onion
½ cup chopped
 ripe tomato
1 dill pickle, sliced
¼ cup shredded
 cheddar cheese

This salad aims to satisfy a craving for fast-food burgers. The shredded lettuce gives it the same texture, while the dressing conveys the flavor of a "special sauce." Add some shredded cheddar and your favorite burger toppings, and you're sure to love this burger-inspired salad.

1. In a medium sauté pan or skillet, brown the ground beef, stirring, for 7 to 10 minutes. Season with the salt and pepper, then drain the meat, if desired.

2. In a small bowl, combine the mayonnaise, ketchup, mustard, and relish.

3. Fill a large bowl with the shredded lettuce. Top with the beef, red onion, tomato, dill pickle, and cheese. Drizzle the dressing over top and serve.

Macronutrients: 75% Fat, 21% Protein, 4% Carbs

Per serving: Calories: 867; Total Fat: 72g; Protein: 45g; Total Carbohydrates: 9g; Fiber: 3g; Erythritol: 0g; Net Carbs: 6g

Greek Salad with Avocado

EGG FREE, NUT FREE, UNDER 30 MINUTES, VEGETARIAN

Serves 4
Prep Time: 10 minutes

This nontraditional take on the classic Greek salad is great for a keto diet; the addition of avocado makes it unique. Also, the crunch and bright flavors of the fresh vegetables contrast nicely with the creamy fat of the avocado. Dress this with homemade Greek dressing, and you've got one amazing salad.

For the salad

3 Roma (plum) tomatoes, seeded and chopped

1 medium cucumber, peeled and cut into ½-inch pieces

1 green bell pepper, cored, seeded, and cut into ½-inch strips

1 cup pitted Kalamata olives

1 medium avocado, cut into ½-inch cubes

½ cup crumbled feta cheese

¼ medium red onion, thinly sliced

For the dressing

1/4 cup extra-virgin olive oil

2 tablespoons red wine vinegar

1 tablespoon chopped fresh parsley

1 garlic clove, minced

1 teaspoon dried oregano

1 teaspoon freshly squeezed lemon juice

½ teaspoon pink Himalayan sea salt

¼ teaspoon freshly ground black pepper

1. **To make the salad:** In a large bowl, combine the tomatoes, cucumber, bell pepper, olives, avocado, feta, and red onion.

2. **To make the dressing:** In a small bowl, combine the olive oil, vinegar, parsley, garlic, oregano, lemon juice, salt, and pepper.

3. Toss the salad ingredients until well coated with the dressing.

Ingredient Tip: When selecting an avocado for this recipe, it is best to go with one that is a little bit on the firmer side. If it's too soft, it won't retain its integrity once the salad is tossed.

Macronutrients: 85% Fat, 7% Protein, 8% Carbs

Per serving: Calories: 334; Total Fat: 31g; Protein: 6g; Total Carbohydrates: 12g; Fiber: 6g; Erythritol: 0g; Net Carbs: 6g

Egg Drop Soup

DAIRY FREE, NUT FREE, ONE POT, UNDER 30 MINUTES

Serves 2
Prep Time: 2 minutes
Cook Time: 10 minutes

4 cups chicken broth

1 teaspoon pink Himalayan
  sea salt

½ teaspoon ground ginger

½ teaspoon toasted
  sesame oil

Pinch of ground
  white pepper

2 large eggs

1 scallion, both white and
  green parts, sliced

This egg drop soup captures the flavor of your favorite Chinese takeout without all the carbs that would normally make it off limits. The broth presents with full flavors of ginger and white pepper, but is still incredibly simple to make.

1. In a medium saucepan, combine the broth, salt, ginger, sesame oil, and white pepper. Cook over medium-high heat until the soup is boiling.

2. In a small bowl, lightly beat the eggs.

3. Stirring the soup in a circular motion, slowly drizzle the beaten egg into the center of the vortex. When all the egg is mixed in, stop stirring.

4. Cook for an additional 2 minutes, until the egg is cooked through, then pour into 2 bowls, sprinkle with the scallions, and serve.

Cooking Tip: This soup is thinner than other egg drop soups you may have had. This is because most restaurants thicken the soup with cornstarch. If you want a similar texture, mix ½ teaspoon xanthan gum with ½ cup water until smooth, then stir it into the soup to thicken it.

Macronutrients: 57% Fat, 32% Protein, 11% Carbs

Per serving: Calories: 121; Total Fat: 8g; Protein: 10g; Total Carbohydrates: 3g; Fiber: 0g; Erythritol: 0g; Net Carbs: 3g

Beef Chili

EGG FREE, NUT FREE, ONE POT

Serves 4
Prep Time: 5 minutes
Cook Time: 50 minutes

½ green bell pepper, cored, seeded, and chopped

½ medium onion, chopped

2 tablespoons extra-virgin olive oil

1 tablespoon minced garlic

1 pound ground beef (80/20)

1 (14-ounce) can crushed tomatoes

1 cup beef broth

1 tablespoon ground cumin

1 tablespoon chili powder

2 teaspoons paprika

1 teaspoon pink Himalayan sea salt

¼ teaspoon cayenne pepper

Whether it's for a cold winter night or a summer barbecue outdoors, chili is the perfect dish. This keto chili doesn't skimp on the flavor, either. It provides a nice balance of heat and acidity, but can be easily modified to fit any taste buds. Serve it in bowls topped with cheese, or spread it on hot dogs to create the perfect keto chili dogs. No matter how you choose to eat it, you won't likely find yourself missing chili again.

1. In a medium pot, combine the bell pepper, onion, and olive oil. Cook over medium heat for 8 to 10 minutes, until the onion is translucent.

2. Add the garlic and cook for 1 minute longer, until fragrant.

3. Add the ground beef and cook for 7 to 10 minutes, until browned.

4. Add the tomatoes, broth, cumin, chili powder, paprika, salt, and cayenne. Stir to combine.

5. Simmer the chili for 30 minutes, until the flavors come together, then enjoy.

Variation Tip: If you allow soy in your keto diet, black soybeans are actually very low in carbs and can be added to this recipe to make it a chili with beans.

Macronutrients: 67% Fat, 23% Protein, 10% Carbs

Per serving: Calories: 406; Total Fat: 31g; Protein: 22g; Total Carbohydrates: 12g; Fiber: 4g; Erythritol: 0g; Net Carbs: 8g

New England Clam Chowder

EGG FREE, NUT FREE, ONE POT

Serves 2
Prep Time: 5 minutes
Cook Time: 25 minutes

2 bacon slices, chopped

1 celery stalk, chopped

¼ medium onion, chopped

1 garlic clove, minced

1 cup chicken broth

2 (6.5-ounce) cans
chopped clams, drained,
juices reserved

1 medium kohlrabi, peeled
and cubed

1 bay leaf

½ teaspoon pink Himalayan
sea salt

¼ teaspoon freshly ground
black pepper

¼ teaspoon dried thyme

Pinch of ground
white pepper

1½ cups heavy
(whipping) cream

This ketogenic take on a New England clam chowder is a game changer. It provides that thick, creamy texture and comforting flavor you know and love, and you don't have to worry about the carb count.

1. In a medium pot, cook the bacon over medium-high heat for 10 to 12 minutes, until crispy. Transfer the bacon to a paper towel–lined plate to cool.

2. In the pot with the bacon grease, sauté the celery and onion for 8 to 10 minutes, until the onion is translucent. Add the garlic and cook for an additional minute, until fragrant.

3. Add the broth, reserved clam juice (not the clams yet), the kohlrabi, bay leaf, salt, black pepper, thyme, and white pepper.

4. Bring to a boil, then reduce the heat to low and simmer for 10 to 15 minutes, until the kohlrabi is tender.

5. Add the cream and clams. Stir to combine.

6. Simmer the soup for roughly 20 minutes, or until it reduces to your desired consistency. Remove and discard the bay leaf.

7. Stir in the bacon crumbles and serve.

Ingredient Tip: If you are unable to find kohlrabi at your grocery store, the next best substitute for potatoes is cauliflower.

Macronutrients: 68% Fat, 23% Protein, 9% Carbs

Per serving: Calories: 939; Total Fat: 73g; Protein: 51g; Total Carbohydrates: 21g; Fiber: 3g; Erythritol: 0g; Net Carbs: 18g

Chicken Noodle Soup

EGG FREE, NUT FREE, ONE POT

Serves 2
Prep Time: 5 minutes
Cook Time: 25 minutes

1 tablespoon extra-virgin
   olive oil
8 ounces boneless, skinless
   chicken thighs, cubed
¼ medium onion, chopped
½ celery stalk, thinly sliced
1 teaspoon minced garlic
2 cups chicken broth
1 teaspoon pink Himalayan
   sea salt
½ teaspoon freshly ground
   black pepper
1 teaspoon dried thyme
1 (7-ounce) package
   shirataki noodles, drained
   (see Tips)

This soup adapts a childhood favorite to your new way of eating. The flavorful broth, tender chicken pieces, and shirataki noodles come together to present the perfect keto chicken noodle soup in a single spoonful.

1. In a large pot, heat the olive oil over medium heat.

2. Cook the chicken for 8 to 10 minutes, until almost cooked through.

3. Add the onion and celery to the pot. Cook for 7 to 10 minutes, until the onion is translucent.

4. Add the garlic and cook for an additional minute, until fragrant.

5. Pour the chicken broth into the pot. Add the salt, pepper, and thyme. Simmer for about 10 minutes to let the flavors develop.

6. Rinse the shirataki noodles, then add them to the pot right before serving.

Ingredient Tip: Shirataki noodles are made from the konjac plant. Miracle Noodles is a widely available brand, but any brand will work. Shirataki noodles can be found in the in the health food section near the noodle alternatives or in the Asian food section.

Variation Tip: If you don't like shirataki noodles, substitute zucchini noodles (zoodles). The texture is slightly different, but equally good.

Macronutrients: 70% Fat, 24% Protein, 6% Carbs

Per serving: Calories: 330; Total Fat: 26g; Protein: 19g; Total Carbohydrates: 5g; Fiber: 0g; Erythritol: 0g; Net Carbs: 5g

Broccoli Cheddar Soup

EGG FREE, NUT FREE, ONE POT, UNDER 30 MINUTES

Serves 2
Prep Time: 5 minutes
Cook Time: 15 minutes

¼ medium onion, chopped

2 tablespoons butter

1 garlic clove, minced

1 cup chicken broth

¾ teaspoon pink Himalayan
   sea salt

½ teaspoon freshly ground
   black pepper

¼ teaspoon dry
   mustard powder

8 ounces fresh broccoli
   florets, cooked and
   finely chopped

1 cup heavy
   (whipping) cream

1 cup shredded
   cheddar cheese

This classic soup could have easily been invented for the keto diet. It combines the nutrients of broccoli with the fat needed to keep you in ketosis. The result is a rich and cheesy soup with a fantastic broccoli flavor.

1. In a medium pot, combine the onion, butter, and garlic over medium heat. Cook for 7 to 10 minutes, until the onion is tender.

2. Add the broth, salt, pepper, and mustard, and bring the mixture to a boil.

3. Reduce the heat and add the broccoli and cream.

4. Slowly add the cheese, stirring.

5. The soup is ready to serve as soon as the cheese is melted and has blended with the rest of the soup.

Macronutrients: 84% Fat, 9% Protein, 7% Carbs

Per serving: Calories: 789; Total Fat: 75g; Protein: 19g; Total Carbohydrates: 14g; Fiber: 4g; Erythritol: 0g; Net Carbs: 10g

Loaded Cauliflower Soup

EGG FREE, NUT FREE, ONE POT

Serves 3
Prep Time: 5 minutes
Cook Time: 25 minutes

2 bacon strips,
   roughly chopped

¼ medium onion, chopped

1½ cups chicken broth

1½ cups chopped
   cauliflower florets

½ teaspoon pink Himalayan
   sea salt

½ teaspoon freshly ground
   black pepper

¼ teaspoon garlic powder

1 cup heavy
   (whipping) cream

1 cup shredded
   cheddar cheese

3 tablespoons sour cream

2 tablespoons chopped
   fresh chives

This is a ketogenic rendition of the classic baked potato soup. It's thick, creamy, and loaded with the flavors of your favorite baked potato toppings. The cauliflower is creamy, smooth, and practically indistinguishable from the potatoes that would traditionally be in this soup. For me this dish is the ultimate comfort food.

1. In a medium saucepan, cook the bacon over medium-high heat for 8 to 10 minutes, until crispy. Transfer the bacon to a paper towel–lined plate.

2. Add the onion to the saucepan and cook for 8 to 10 minutes, until tender.

3. Add the broth, cauliflower, salt, pepper, and garlic powder. Bring to a simmer and cook for about 5 minutes, until the cauliflower is tender.

4. Reduce the heat and stir in the cream. Slowly stir in the cheese.

5. Divide the soup among 3 serving bowls. Top each bowl with 1 tablespoon of sour cream and equal portions of the bacon crumbles and chives.

Variation Tip: Kohlrabi is a great substitute for potatoes. To put a little different spin on this soup, try using kohlrabi instead of the cauliflower.

Macronutrients: 84% Fat, 11% Protein, 5% Carbs

Per serving: Calories: 510; Total Fat: 48g; Protein: 15g; Total Carbohydrates: 7g; Fiber: 1g; Erythritol: 0g; Net Carbs: 6g

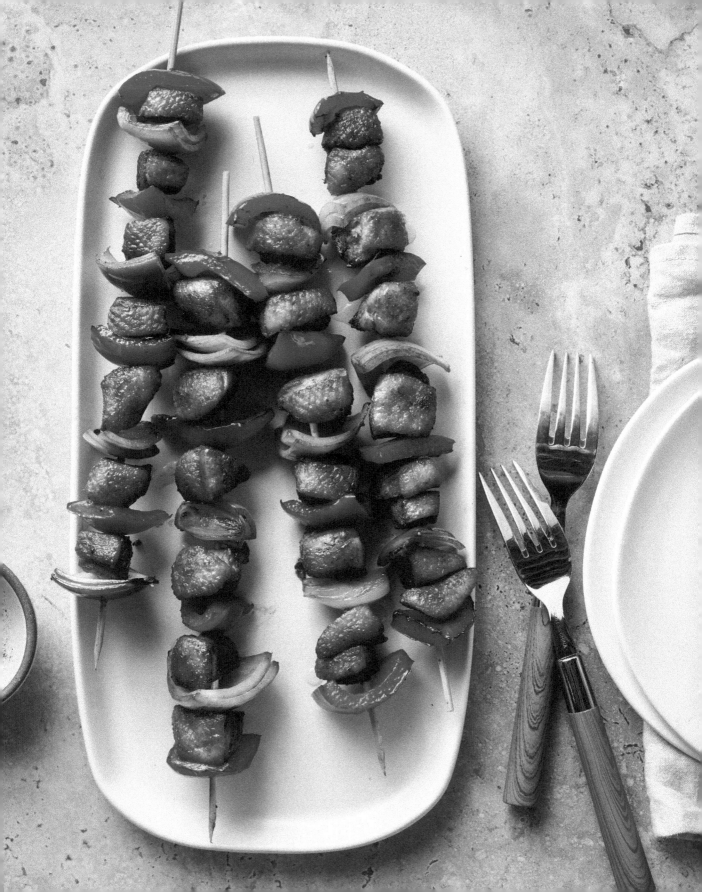

CHAPTER FIVE

Poultry

Chicken Alfredo

EGG FREE, NUT FREE, UNDER 30 MINUTES

Serves 2
Prep Time: 5 minutes
Cook Time: 20 minutes

2 teaspoons extra-virgin
  olive oil, divided
8 ounces boneless, skinless
  chicken thighs, cubed
2 tablespoons butter
½ teaspoon minced garlic
½ cup heavy
  (whipping) cream
⅔ cup grated
  Parmesan cheese
¼ cup shredded
  low-moisture
  mozzarella cheese
Pinch of red pepper flakes
Pink Himalayan sea salt
Freshly ground
  black pepper
1 (7-ounce) package
  shirataki noodles,
  drained, or 7 ounces
  zoodles (spiralized
  zucchini)

When it comes to pasta dishes, fettuccini Alfredo has always been one of my favorites. So, when I started a keto diet, this was one of the first dishes I adapted. The sauce is the star of the show, rich with the flavors of garlic and Parmesan cheese. Pour this amazing sauce over your favorite keto pasta substitute, and you'll never miss Alfredo again.

1. In a small sauté pan or skillet, heat 1 teaspoon of olive oil over medium heat and cook the chicken for 10 to 12 minutes, until cooked through.

2. In a medium saucepan, melt the butter over medium heat. Add the garlic and cook for 1 to 2 minutes, until slightly browned. Add the cream and bring to a simmer.

3. Slowly add the Parmesan and mozzarella while stirring. The cheese should melt into the sauce.

4. Reduce the heat, add the chicken, and heat through, without allowing the sauce to boil. Season with the salt and pepper.

5. In the same skillet as you cooked the chicken, add the remaining 1 teaspoon of olive oil and drop in the shirataki noodles. Cook the noodles over medium heat for 2 to 3 minutes, until heated through.

6. Spoon the noodles onto 2 serving plates and top with the sauce.

Macronutrients: 76% Fat, 18% Protein, 6% Carbs

Per serving: Calories: 810; Total Fat: 70g; Protein: 36g; Total Carbohydrates: 11g; Fiber: 2g; Erythritol: 0g; Net Carbs: 9g

Chicken Cordon Bleu

EGG FREE, NUT FREE

Serves 2
Prep Time: 10 minutes
Cook Time: 25 minutes

For the chicken

2 tablespoons grated
   Parmesan cheese

¼ cup pork panko crumbs
   or finely ground fried
   pork rinds (see Tip)

1 teaspoon extra-virgin
   olive oil

½ teaspoon garlic powder

½ teaspoon onion powder

½ teaspoon pink Himalayan
   sea salt

¼ teaspoon freshly ground
   black pepper

2 large boneless, skinless
   chicken thighs

4 thin slices Swiss cheese

4 ounces thin deli
   ham slices

Ingredient List Continues ▸

If you've never cooked chicken cordon bleu, then you're missing out on something magical. Traditionally it's a breaded chicken cutlet (I use boneless, skinless thighs) stuffed with ham and loaded with Swiss cheese. Once baked, it is topped with a creamy, tangy sauce that makes for an unforgettable dish.

1. Preheat the oven to 425°F. Position a baking rack on a baking sheet.

2. **To make the chicken:** In a food processor, pulse together the Parmesan, pork crumbs, olive oil, garlic powder, onion powder, salt, and pepper. Place the mixture in a shallow dish.

3. Open up the chicken thighs, and flatten them as much as possible. Sandwich each piece between 2 sheets of plastic wrap. Using a meat hammer or a rolling pin, pound the chicken to a thickness of about ½ inch.

4. Lay the chicken pieces on a work surface. Place half the cheese and half the ham on each cutlet.

5. Roll the chicken pieces into a cylinder, encasing the cheese and ham, and secure with a toothpick.

6. Dip the chicken in the breading, generously covering each roll and patting on additional crumbs to coat well.

7. Place the chicken rolls on the baking rack.

8. Bake for 15 to 20 minutes, until an instant-read thermometer inserted into the center of a roll reads 165°F and the juices run clear when the chicken is pierced.

CONTINUES ▸

Chicken Cordon Bleu CONTINUED

For the sauce

1 tablespoon butter

1 garlic clove, minced

½ cup chicken broth

½ cup heavy
  (whipping) cream

1 tablespoon Dijon mustard

½ cup grated
  Parmesan cheese

Pink Himalayan sea salt

Freshly ground
  black pepper

9. **To make the sauce:** In a medium saucepan, heat the butter and garlic over medium heat for 2 to 3 minutes, until the mixture begins to brown.

10. Add the broth, cream, and mustard and bring to a simmer.

11. Stir in the Parmesan and continue to simmer, stirring, until the cheese is melted and the sauce is reduced to your desired consistency.

12. Season the sauce with salt and pepper.

13. Transfer the chicken rolls to plates and top with the sauce.

> **Ingredient Tip:** You can find pork panko crumbs at Asian markets, if you don't want to create them yourself by grinding fried pork rinds in a food processor.

Macronutrients: 64% Fat, 31% Protein, 5% Carbs

Per serving: Calories: 1016; Total Fat: 72g; Protein: 80g; Total Carbohydrates: 12g; Fiber: 2g; Erythritol: 0g; Net Carbs: 10g

Chicken Parmesan

EGG FREE, NUT FREE

Serves 4
Prep Time: 10 minutes
Cook Time: 20 minutes

For the chicken

2 tablespoons extra-virgin
olive oil, plus more for
greasing

2 ounces (½ cup) pork
panko crumbs or finely
ground fried pork rinds

¼ cup grated
Parmesan cheese

½ teaspoon Italian
seasoning

½ teaspoon pink Himalayan
sea salt

¼ teaspoon freshly ground
black pepper

4 boneless, skinless
chicken thighs

½ cup shredded
low-moisture
mozzarella cheese

Ingredient List Continues ▶

This dish is perfect for any night of the week. The chicken has a slightly crisp breading made from Parmesan cheese and pork panko crumbs, and it is topped with a garlic marinara sauce. Crown this with some gooey mozzarella, and you're in for a real treat. You might even find yourself going back for seconds, so this recipe intentionally makes four servings.

1. **To make the chicken:** Preheat the oven to 450°F. Grease a baking sheet with a little olive oil.

2. In a food processor, combine the pork crumbs, Parmesan, Italian seasoning, salt, and pepper. Pulse until the crumbs are very fine. Transfer to a shallow dish.

3. In another shallow dish, spread the 2 tablespoons olive oil.

4. Pat the chicken thighs dry with a paper towel. Dip them in the olive oil, coating both sides.

5. Dip the chicken in the breading, patting on additional crumbs so the pieces are generously coated. Place the chicken on the baking sheet.

6. Bake for 12 to 14 minutes, until an instant-read thermometer inserted into the center of a chicken thigh reads 165°F and the juices run clear when the chicken is pierced. (If an extra-crispy coating on the chicken is desired, transfer the chicken to the broiler for a minute or so to crisp the breading further.)

CONTINUES ▶

Chicken Parmesan CONTINUED

For the sauce

¼ cup tomato puree

½ teaspoon minced garlic

¼ teaspoon Italian seasoning

¼ teaspoon pink Himalayan sea salt

7. **To make the sauce:** In a small bowl, combine the tomato puree, garlic, Italian seasoning, and salt.

8. Top each chicken thigh with 1 tablespoon of the tomato sauce and 2 tablespoons of the mozzarella.

9. Bake (in the oven) for 5 more minutes, until the cheese is melted. Transfer the chicken to individual plates and serve.

Storage Tip: Store any leftover sauce in an airtight container in the refrigerator for 3 to 5 days.

Macronutrients: 69% Fat, 29% Protein, 2% Carbs

Per serving: Calories: 628; Total Fat: 48g; Protein: 45g; Total Carbohydrates: 4g; Fiber: 0g; Erythritol: 0g; Net Carbs: 4g

Crunchy Chicken Tacos

EGG FREE, NUT FREE

Serves 4
Prep Time: 5 minutes
Cook Time: 30 minutes to 8 hours

1 pound frozen boneless, skinless chicken thighs

1 cup chicken broth

1 cup low-carb green salsa (see Tip)

½ medium onion, chopped

2 teaspoons minced garlic

8 slices provolone cheese

1 cup shredded lettuce

¼ cup chopped ripe tomato

½ cup sour cream

This recipe makes use of the same techniques used to produce cheese crisps in order to create a delicious, crunchy taco shell. The chicken filling is tender and loaded with flavor. It has a mild heat that is offset by the accompanying lettuce, tomato, and sour cream. You'll need a slow cooker or pressure cooker for this recipe.

1. In a slow cooker or electric pressure cooker, combine the chicken thighs, broth, salsa, onion, and garlic.

2. Place the lid on the pot. If using a slow cooker, cook on the low setting for 7 to 8 hours or on high for 3 to 4 hours. If using a pressure cooker, cook for 20 minutes on high pressure, then quick-release the pressure.

3. Place a slice of the provolone on a piece of parchment paper (not wax paper). Microwave on high power for 45 seconds; the cheese should just begin to turn a brownish orange in a few spots.

4. Quickly and carefully remove the parchment paper from the microwave. Holding opposite edges of the paper, form the melted cheese into a U shape. Hold it in this position for about 10 seconds, until it cools enough to hold its shape. (You can also hang the microwaved cheese slice over a wooden spoon handle to form the shape.) Remove the taco from the parchment paper. Repeat with the remaining 7 cheese slices.

5. Using a slotted spoon, remove the chicken from the cooker. Using 2 forks, shred the chicken, then return it to the cooker.

CONTINUES ▶

6. Use tongs or a slotted spoon to fill the tacos with equal portions of the chicken, being careful to drain off some of the liquid so the tacos don't get soggy.

7. Top the chicken filling with shredded lettuce, tomato, and sour cream, then serve.

Ingredient Tip: When looking for green salsa, watch out for sugar on the ingredient label. At my local store, there are only two brands that do not contain sugar.

Macronutrients: 67% Fat, 28% Protein, 5% Carbs

Per serving: Calories: 528; Total Fat: 40g; Protein: 35g; Total Carbohydrates: 8g; Fiber: 2g; Erythritol: 0g; Net Carbs: 6g

Teriyaki Chicken

DAIRY FREE, EGG FREE, NUT FREE, ONE PAN, UNDER 30 MINUTES

Serves 2
Prep Time: 5 minutes
Cook Time: 20 minutes

⅓ cup coconut aminos or
   soy sauce
2 tablespoons brown
   erythritol
2 tablespoons allulose
1 tablespoon sesame seeds
¼ teaspoon freshly ground
   black pepper
1 teaspoon extra-virgin
   olive oil
1 pound boneless, skinless
   chicken thighs, cut into
   1-inch cubes
1 (8-ounce) package
   cauliflower rice, cooked
1 scallion, green part only,
   thinly sliced

Teriyaki chicken is one of my favorite dishes. The challenge in making it keto is creating that sweet, syrupy sauce without any sugar. Thanks to a new ingredient called allulose, this was possible. The dish tastes just like it's made with the traditional teriyaki sauce that everyone knows and loves.

1. In a small bowl, combine the coconut aminos, brown erythritol, allulose, sesame seeds, and pepper.

2. In a medium sauté pan or skillet, heat the olive oil over medium heat. Add the chicken and stir quickly. Cook the chicken for 10 to 12 minutes, until all sides are nicely browned and the chicken is no longer pink in the middle.

3. Add the sauce and stir with a rubber scraper. The liquid will begin to bubble rapidly. Reduce the sauce for about 5 minutes, until it's thick and syrupy.

4. Serve over the cauliflower rice. Garnish with the scallion greens.

Ingredient Tip: Allulose, much like erythritol, is not absorbed by the body. For this reason, it can be subtracted from your net carbs on a keto diet. The total carbs from allulose must appear on the nutrition label of packing as a carb, but it does not affect blood sugar. See allulose.org for more information.

Macronutrients: 64% Fat, 30% Protein, 6% Carbs

Per serving: Calories: 599; Total Fat: 43g; Protein: 44g; Total Carbohydrates: 9g; Fiber: 3g; Erythritol: 12g; Allulose: 12g; Net Carbs: 6g

Chicken Pot Pie

Serves 4
Prep Time: 20 minutes
Cook Time: 25 minutes

For the filling

½ medium onion, chopped

2 celery stalks, chopped

½ cup fresh or frozen peas

2 tablespoons butter

1 garlic clove, minced

1½ pounds boneless,
  skinless chicken thighs,
  cut into 1-inch cubes

1 cup chicken broth

½ cup heavy
  (whipping) cream

½ cup shredded
  low-moisture
  mozzarella cheese

1 teaspoon dried thyme

½ teaspoon pink Himalayan
  sea salt

½ teaspoon freshly ground
  black pepper

This chicken pot pie has a creamy and flavorful filling that tastes as great as it smells when baking in the oven. The crust is light, buttery, and flaky. With this recipe, you'll never miss a traditional chicken pot pie again!

1. **To make the filling:** In a large saucepan, combine the onion, celery, peas, butter, and garlic over medium heat. Cook for 3 to 5 minutes, until the onion starts to turn translucent.

2. In a large skillet, cook the chicken thighs for 3 to 5 minutes, until there is no more visible pink. Add the cooked chicken and all juices to the pan with the vegetables.

3. Add the broth, cream, mozzarella, thyme, salt, and pepper to the pan. Simmer over medium heat for 5 minutes, until the sauce thickens, stirring occasionally.

4. Preheat the oven to 400°F.

5. **To make the crust:** In a medium bowl, combine the almond flour, butter, sour cream, egg white, flaxseed, xanthan gum, baking powder, garlic powder, salt, and thyme. Mix well, forming the dough into a ball.

6. Place the dough between 2 sheets of parchment paper and roll out into a 10-inch round that is ¼ inch thick.

7. Fill an 8-inch pie pan or 4 (6-ounce) ramekins with the chicken filling.

For the crust

1 cup almond flour

2 tablespoons butter, at room temperature

2 tablespoons sour cream

1 large egg white

1 tablespoon ground flaxseed

1 teaspoon xanthan gum

1 teaspoon baking powder

½ teaspoon garlic powder

¼ teaspoon pink Himalayan sea salt

¼ teaspoon dried thyme

8. Top the pie pan with the crust, flipping it onto the filling and the peeling away the parchment paper. If using ramekins, cut circles of the dough and fit them onto the ramekins. Pinch to seal the edges, and trim off any excess. Pierce the top of the crust with a fork to create steam holes.

9. Bake for 10 to 12 minutes, until the crust is lightly browned.

10. Let cool for 5 minutes, then serve.

Macronutrients: 73% Fat, 20% Protein, 6% Carbs

Per serving: Calories: 817; Total Fat: 68g; Protein: 41g; Total Carbohydrates: 13g; Fiber: 5g; Erythritol: 0g; Net Carbs: 8g

Jalapeño Cheddar Chicken Casserole

EGG FREE, NUT FREE

Serves 2
Prep Time: 10 minutes
Cook Time: 35 minutes

1 tablespoon extra-virgin
   olive oil
1 pound boneless, skinless
   chicken thighs, cut into
   ½-inch cubes
4 ounces full-fat
   cream cheese
2 jalapeño peppers,
   sliced, seeds and
   membranes removed
¼ cup heavy
   (whipping) cream
¼ cup chicken broth
½ teaspoon pink Himalayan
   sea salt
¼ teaspoon garlic powder
¼ teaspoon onion powder
½ cup shredded cheddar
   cheese, divided
1 cup cooked
   cauliflower rice

There's something about jalapeño and chicken that makes them go together in an amazing way. This casserole highlights these flavors while pairing them with the sharpness of cheddar and the creaminess of cream cheese. The cauliflower rice lends some substance and texture. This simple dish is one you'll want to keep in your regular rotation.

1. Preheat the oven to 375°F.
2. In a medium sauté pan or skillet, heat the olive oil over medium-high heat and add the chicken. Cook for 10 to 12 minutes, until the chicken is no longer pink.
3. In a medium saucepan, combine the cream cheese, jalapeños, cream, broth, salt, garlic powder, and onion powder over medium heat. Stir until the cream cheese melts into the sauce. Add ¼ cup of cheddar cheese, and continue to stir until it melts into the sauce.
4. In an 8-inch square baking dish, combine the chicken and cauliflower rice.
5. Pour in the cheese sauce, then sprinkle the remaining ¼ cup of cheddar cheese over the top.
6. Bake for 20 minutes, until the sauce is bubbling. Let cool for 10 minutes, then serve.

Macronutrients: 76% Fat, 21% Protein, 3% Carbs

Per serving: Calories: 994; Total Fat: 85g; Protein: 50g; Total Carbohydrates: 9g; Fiber: 2g; Erythritol: 0g; Net Carbs: 7g

Jamaican Jerk Chicken

DAIRY FREE, EGG FREE, NUT FREE

Serves 4
Prep Time: 10 minutes,
plus 12 hours to marinate
Cook Time: 45 minutes

¼ medium white onion
¼ cup extra-virgin olive oil
1 to 3 habanero chiles
2 tablespoons granulated
    erythritol
2 tablespoons jerk
    seasoning
1 tablespoon coconut
    aminos or soy sauce
Juice of 1 lime
1 tablespoon minced garlic
4 chicken leg quarters
    (thighs and drumsticks)
2 scallions, white and
    green parts, sliced

Inspired by an unbelievable food tasting experience in the Caribbean, this ketogenic take on a Jamaican jerk chicken is a guaranteed way to spice up your lunch or dinner. Depending on your preference, the chicken can be toned down to a mild amount of heat or turned up to blazing. Don't let the spices fool you—this chicken is juicy, crispy, and loaded with flavors of the island. I prefer to make jerk chicken on the grill because it adds color, but baking in the oven also creates a succulent dish. Note that you need to start this preparation 12 to 24 hours ahead.

1. In a food processor, combine the onion, olive oil, chiles, erythritol, jerk seasoning, coconut aminos, lime juice, and garlic. Puree on high until the mixture is smooth. Transfer this marinade to a resealable 1-gallon plastic bag.

2. Add the chicken to the bag, then seal and shake the bag until the chicken is well coated with the seasoning. Allow to marinate in the refrigerator for 12 to 24 hours, preferably 24.

3. Set a grill to high or preheat the oven to 425°F.

4. Remove the chicken from the marinade bag and place it on the grill or on a rack set on a baking sheet. Reserve the marinade. Cook the chicken for 30 to 35 minutes, flipping the pieces every 15 minutes. An instant-read thermometer inserted between the thigh and drumstick should read 165°F, and the juices should run clear when the chicken is pierced.

CONTINUES ▶

5. Transfer the marinade to a small saucepan and set it over high heat. Cook for about 10 minutes, or until it reaches just over 165°F.

6. Place the chicken on a serving platter. Top with the scallions and serve with the jerk sauce on the side.

Cooking Tip: When handling habanero chiles, it is best to wear protective gloves, as the juices can irritate your skin. Wearing gloves is also a reminder to avoid touching your eyes or face.

Storage Tip: Leftovers make this a great lunch for the next day. Any uneaten portions should be stored in an airtight container in your refrigerator for up to 4 days.

Macronutrients: 70% Fat, 28% Protein, 2% Carbs

Per serving: Calories: 884; Total Fat: 68g; Protein: 58g; Total Carbohydrates: 7g; Fiber: 1g; Erythritol: 6g; Net Carbs: 6g

Crispy Chicken Tenders

Serves 2
Prep Time: 10 minutes
Cook Time: 25 minutes

Coconut oil cooking spray
¼ cup almond flour
¼ cup grated
  Parmesan cheese
½ teaspoon pink Himalayan
  sea salt
½ teaspoon onion powder
¼ teaspoon garlic powder
¼ teaspoon freshly ground
  black pepper
Pinch of ground
  white pepper
1 large egg
1 pound boneless, skinless
  chicken thighs, cut into
  ½-inch-wide strips
Ranch dressing (optional)

A dish loved by adults and children alike, chicken tenders have become an American favorite. This preparation brings the crunchy texture and peppery flavor of the familiar chicken tenders to a ketogenic diet. Dip the finished pieces in some ranch dressing to add extra fat, and you'll finally enjoy chicken tenders on your keto diet.

1. Preheat the oven to 350°F. Place a baking rack on a baking sheet, then spray the rack with cooking spray.
2. On a large plate, combine the almond flour, Parmesan, salt, onion powder, garlic powder, black pepper, and white pepper.
3. In a small bowl, lightly beat the egg.
4. Dip each chicken strip into the egg, shaking off any excess, and then roll the chicken in the flour mixture, again shaking off any excess.
5. Place the chicken strips on the baking rack, then lightly spray the tops of the strips with a little more cooking spray.
6. Bake for 15 to 20 minutes.
7. Turn on the broiler on high and broil the chicken strips for 3 to 4 minutes, until golden brown and crispy. Serve with ranch dressing, if desired.

Variation Tip: You can also use this same recipe to make true chicken breast tenders; they will just be a little bit lower in fat. The thighs offer more fat, and for this reason it is worthwhile to slice your own chicken thighs.

Macronutrients: 43% Fat, 53% Protein, 4% Carbs

Per serving: Calories: 433; Total Fat: 21g; Protein: 54g; Total Carbohydrates: 5g; Fiber: 2g; Erythritol: 0g; Net Carbs: 3g

Turkey with Mushroom Gravy

EGG FREE, NUT FREE

Serves 4
Prep Time: 10 minutes
Cook Time: 45 minutes

1 (2-pound) piece of
turkey breast
½ teaspoon pink Himalayan
sea salt, plus more for
seasoning
¼ teaspoon freshly ground
black pepper, plus more
for seasoning
4 tablespoons
(½ stick) butter
2 cups sliced fresh
mushrooms
½ medium onion, chopped
1 cup chicken broth
¼ cup sour cream

When it comes to keeping a ketogenic diet, making turkey dishes can be tricky because turkey is a lean meat. In this case, the turkey is smothered with a delicious sour cream, onion, and mushroom gravy. The turkey breast remains juicy, each bite coated with creamy gravy and accompanied by tender mushrooms.

1. Preheat the oven to 450°F.

2. Slice the turkey breast into 4 cutlets that are roughly 2 inches thick.

3. Place the cutlets in an 8-inch square baking dish and season lightly with a little salt and pepper. Bake for 30 minutes.

4. In a medium saucepan, melt the butter over medium heat. Add the mushrooms and onion and cook for 3 to 5 minutes, until the onion is almost translucent.

5. Add the broth, sour cream, ½ teaspoon of salt, and ¼ teaspoon of pepper to the pan. Stir to form a sauce, then simmer over low heat for about 5 minutes, until it reaches your desired thickness. Keep warm.

6. When the turkey is almost finished baking, pour the gravy over it and bake for an additional 5 to 10 minutes, until the gravy is bubbling. Serve.

Macronutrients: 54% Fat, 44% Protein, 2% Carbs

Per serving: Calories: 499; Total Fat: 30g; Protein: 51g; Total Carbohydrates: 3g; Fiber: 1g; Erythritol: 0g; Net Carbs: 2g

Duck Shish Kebab

DAIRY FREE, EGG FREE, NUT FREE

Serves 2
Prep Time: 10 minutes
Cook Time: 20 minutes

2 boneless, skin-on
duck breasts, cut into
1-inch cubes

1 teaspoon Chinese
five-spice powder

¼ teaspoon pink Himalayan
sea salt

¼ teaspoon freshly ground
black pepper

1 red bell pepper, cored,
seeded, and cut into
1-inch chunks

½ small red onion, cut into
1-inch slices and then
quartered

1 teaspoon extra-virgin
olive oil

Duck and Chinese five-spice powder go together like peanut butter and jelly—the flavors complement each other perfectly. Here the duck is skewered with pieces of onion and bell pepper. As it cooks, the meat absorbs some of these flavor notes as well, becoming juicy and delicious.

1. If using bamboo skewers, soak them in water for 30 minutes. Preheat the oven to 350°F. Line a baking sheet with parchment paper.

2. In a large bowl, sprinkle the duck cubes with the five-spice powder, salt, and pepper. Toss the duck to evenly distribute the seasonings.

3. Using metal or bamboo skewers, alternate pieces of bell pepper, duck, and onion, then repeat. Keep the fat side of the duck cubes facing outward in the same direction.

4. In a large sauté pan or skillet, heat the olive oil over medium-high heat.

5. Place the skewers in the skillet and cook for about 1 minute on each side, except the fat side. Cook the fat side for 2 to 3 minutes. The skewers should be browned on all sides.

6. Transfer the skewers to the baking sheet and bake for 15 to 20 minutes, until the duck is cooked through and the vegetables are tender. Serve.

Macronutrients: 62% Fat, 31% Protein, 7% Carbs

Per serving: Calories: 297; Total Fat: 21g; Protein: 22g; Total Carbohydrates: 5g; Fiber: 2g; Erythritol: 0g; Net Carbs: 3g

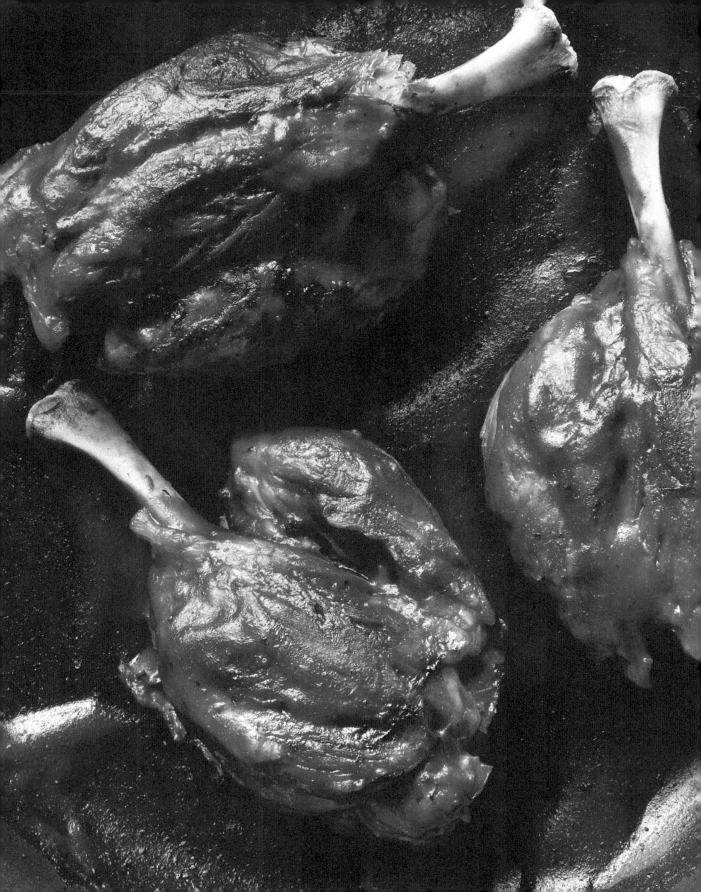

CHAPTER SIX

Meat

Cheesy Meatloaf

NUT FREE

Serves 3
Prep Time: 10 minutes
Cook Time: 60 minutes

This ketogenic take on meatloaf combines all the flavors you love and expect, plus loads of cheese. The meatloaf is tender and juicy, with a fantastic fat content. If you're craving that nostalgic taste, then you've found it here.

For the meatloaf

Butter, for greasing

1 pound ground
   beef (80/20)

½ cup grated
   Parmesan cheese

¼ medium onion, chopped

1 large egg

1 tablespoon
   sugar-free ketchup

1 garlic clove, minced

1 teaspoon coconut aminos
   or soy sauce

1 teaspoon dried parsley

½ teaspoon pink Himalayan
   sea salt

¼ teaspoon freshly ground
   black pepper

For the sauce

¼ cup sugar-free ketchup

1 tablespoon powdered
   erythritol

1. **To make the meatloaf:** Preheat the oven to 350°F. Coat an 8-inch loaf pan with some butter.

2. In a large bowl, combine the beef, Parmesan, onion, egg, ketchup, garlic, coconut aminos, parsley, salt, and pepper. Using your hands, mix the ingredients until well blended.

3. Transfer the mixture to the loaf pan and shape into a loaf, leveling the top with your hand or a rubber spatula.

4. **To make the sauce:** In a small bowl, combine the ketchup and erythritol, mixing until the erythritol has dissolved.

5. Pour the sauce onto the meatloaf, spreading it evenly across the top.

6. Bake for 55 to 60 minutes, until an instant-read thermometer inserted in the center of the meatloaf reaches 160°F and no pink remains. Let the meatloaf cool for 10 to 15 minutes, then slice and serve.

Variation Tip: This recipe can easily be made barbecue style by replacing the ketchup with a sugar-free barbecue sauce.

Macronutrients: 68% Fat, 29% Protein, 3% Carbs

Per serving: Calories: 492; Total Fat: 37g; Protein: 33g; Total Carbohydrates: 4g; Fiber: 0g; Erythritol: 5g; Net Carbs: 4g

Braised Short Ribs

EGG FREE, NUT FREE

Serves 2
Prep Time: 15 minutes
Cook Time: 2 hours
30 minutes

2 tablespoons butter

4 bone-in beef chuck short
  ribs (about 2 pounds)

Pink Himalayan sea salt

Freshly ground
  black pepper

1 garlic clove

2 sprigs fresh thyme

1 sprig fresh rosemary

1½ cups beef broth

1½ cups red wine

These braised short ribs are fall-off-the-bone tender and infused with the flavors of garlic and rosemary. Slow braising them with red wine and herbs creates a fragrant sauce that is reduced before serving. The high fat levels in beef short ribs make this a perfect keto meal.

1. Preheat the oven to 350°F.

2. In a large sauté pan or skillet, melt the butter over medium heat.

3. Season the ribs on all sides with salt and pepper.

4. Add the ribs to the skillet, sear on both sides for 4 to 6 minutes, until uniformly browned.

5. Transfer the ribs to an 8-inch baking pan; leave the drippings in the skillet.

6. Add the garlic, thyme, and rosemary to the skillet and stir for 2 to 3 minutes, until the garlic is browned.

7. Add the broth and wine, and stir to combine. Simmer over low heat until the liquid is reduced by about one-fourth.

8. Pour the sauce over the short ribs and cover the baking pan with aluminum foil. Bake for 2½ hours, until the ribs are very tender.

9. Using a slotted spoon or a fork, transfer the ribs to a serving dish. Pour the cooking liquid through a mesh strainer into a medium bowl. Discard the solids. Drizzle a small amount of the strained liquid over the ribs before serving.

Macronutrients: 75% Fat, 24% Protein, 1% Carbs

Per serving: Calories: 696; Total Fat: 55g; Protein: 39g; Total Carbohydrates: 2g; Fiber: 0g; Erythritol: 0g; Net Carbs: 2g

Beef Barbacoa

DAIRY FREE, EGG FREE, NUT FREE

Serves 4
Prep Time: 20 minutes
Cook Time: 3 hours

1 cup beef broth

½ cup tomato puree

¼ cup granulated erythritol

¼ cup chili powder

2 tablespoons freshly
squeezed lime juice

2 dried chipotle
chiles, crushed

2 tablespoons apple
cider vinegar

4 garlic cloves, minced

1 teaspoon dried oregano

1 teaspoon ground cumin

½ teaspoon pink Himalayan
sea salt

¼ teaspoon freshly ground
black pepper

⅛ teaspoon ground
cinnamon

⅛ teaspoon ground allspice

⅛ teaspoon ground cloves

1½ pounds boneless
chuck roast

2 bay leaves

4 low-carb tortillas

Taco toppings of choice

Beef barbacoa combines shredded tender beef with a sweet, smoky sauce. Typically served in a tortilla, this preparation is best described as a spicy barbecued beef taco. When accompanied by your favorite taco toppings, it is perfect for your Taco Tuesday—or any other day of the week. You'll need a slow cooker for this recipe.

1. In a large bowl, combine the broth, tomato puree, erythritol, chili powder, lime juice, chipotles, vinegar, garlic, oregano, cumin, salt, pepper, cinnamon, allspice, and cloves.

2. If you wish to have a super-smooth sauce and don't mind the added dishes, transfer the mixture to a food processor and run on high speed until the sauce is smooth.

3. Place the chuck roast into a slow cooker. Add the bay leaves and pour in the sauce.

4. Cover and cook on high power for 3 to 4 hours.

5. Remove the inner pot from the slow cooker and discard the bay leaves. Using 2 forks, shred the beef.

6. Pile the barbecued beef into the tortillas, and serve along with your favorite taco toppings.

> **Storage Tip:** This meal makes a great meal prep for the week. Store any leftovers in an airtight container in your refrigerator for 4 to 5 days, then simply reheat a portion and add your toppings.

Macronutrients: 58% Fat, 30% Protein, 12% Carbs

Per serving: Calories: 528; Total Fat: 34g; Protein: 40g; Total Carbohydrates: 30g; Fiber: 19g; Erythritol: 12g; Net Carbs: 11g

Cottage Pie

EGG FREE, NUT FREE

Serves 4
Prep Time: 20 minutes
Cook Time: 30 minutes

For the pie

2 tablespoons extra-virgin
olive oil

2 celery stalks, chopped

½ medium onion, chopped

2 garlic cloves, minced

1 pound ground
beef (80/20)

¼ cup chicken broth

1 tablespoon tomato paste

1 teaspoon pink Himalayan
sea salt

1 teaspoon freshly ground
black pepper

½ teaspoon ground
white pepper

For the topping

2 (12-ounce) packages
cauliflower rice, cooked
and drained

1 cup shredded
low-moisture
mozzarella cheese

The traditional English dish of shepherd's pie is the ultimate comfort food for me. This cottage pie is pretty much the same thing, but made with beef instead of lamb. The filling is both hearty and full of flavor, and the mashed cauliflower topping offers a creamy alternative to the usual mashed potatoes. This might be the perfect meal for a cold winter night.

1. Preheat the oven to 400°F.

2. **To make the pie:** In a large sauté pan or skillet, heat the olive oil over medium heat. Add the celery and onion and cook for 8 to 10 minutes, until the onion is tender.

3. Add the garlic and cook for an additional minute, until fragrant.

4. Add the ground beef, breaking it up with a wooden spoon or spatula. Continue to cook the beef for 7 to 10 minutes, until fully browned.

5. Stir in the broth and tomato paste and stir to coat the meat. Sprinkle in the salt, black pepper, and white pepper.

6. Transfer the meat mixture to a 9-by-13-inch baking dish.

7. **To make the topping:** In a food processor, combine the cauliflower rice, mozzarella, cream, butter, salt, black pepper, white pepper, and garlic powder. Puree on high speed until the mixture is smooth, scraping down the sides of the bowl as necessary.

2 tablespoons heavy
  (whipping) cream

2 tablespoons butter

½ teaspoon pink Himalayan
  sea salt

½ teaspoon freshly ground
  black pepper

¼ teaspoon ground
  white pepper

¼ teaspoon garlic powder

8. Spread the cauliflower mash over the top of the meat and smooth the top.

9. Bake for 10 minutes, until the topping is just lightly browned. Let cool for 5 minutes, then serve.

Variation Tip: If you want to make a shepherd's pie, swap the beef for some ground lamb. Also, add a pinch of rosemary and thyme to complement the flavors.

Macronutrients: 70% Fat, 21% Protein, 9% Carbs

Per serving: Calories: 564; Total Fat: 44g; Protein: 30g; Total Carbohydrates: 13g; Fiber: 4g; Erythritol: 0g; Net Carbs: 7g

Garlic Steak Bites

EGG FREE, NUT FREE, ONE PAN, UNDER 30 MINUTES

Serves 2
Prep Time: 5 minutes
Cook Time: 15 minutes

1 tablespoon beef tallow
   (see Tip)
1 pound boneless
   chuck steak, cut into
   1-inch cubes
Pink Himalayan sea salt
Freshly ground
   black pepper
3 tablespoons butter
2 garlic cloves, minced
½ teaspoon dried rosemary

Steak is a frequent meal in my house. I can't get enough of that golden-brown crust on a perfectly cooked cut of beef. With these steak bites, that same crispy crust is on as much surface area as possible, transforming a simple chuck steak into an incredibly flavorful and affordable cut of meat.

1. In a large sauté pan or skillet, melt the tallow over medium-high heat.

2. Season the steak cubes with salt and pepper on all sides. Add the steak cubes to the pan.

3. Cook on all sides, turning and stirring, for 30 seconds to 1 minute per side. You're just trying to build a nice crust. Transfer the meat to a bowl; leave the drippings in the skillet.

4. Add the butter, garlic, and rosemary to the drippings. Cook over medium heat for 2 to 3 minutes, until the garlic starts to brown.

5. Return the steak to the skillet, and cook, stirring occasionally, for 5 to 10 minutes, until the pieces reach your desired doneness. Check the internal temperature with an instant-read thermometer; I like to cook the meat to 135°F for medium-rare.

Variation Tip: I use chuck steak here to show that affordable steak can still taste great, but if you have a little room in your budget, try this preparation with a rib eye steak.

Ingredient Tip: Tallow is essentially a rendered form of beef fat. It is fantastic for adding a crust to steaks. You'll typically find it in the fats and oils section of your grocery store. It is usually near the ghee and lard. If you cannot find tallow, any other high-smoking-point oil or fat will work.

Macronutrients: 76% Fat, 23% Protein, 1% Carbs

Per serving: Calories: 730; Total Fat: 62g; Protein: 43g; Total Carbohydrates: 1g; Fiber: 0g; Erythritol: 0g; Net Carbs: 1g

Pepper Steak Stir-Fry

DAIRY FREE, EGG FREE, NUT FREE, ONE PAN

Serves 3
Prep Time: 10 minutes
Cook Time: 20 minutes

1 tablespoon extra-virgin
   olive oil, or more
   as needed
1 red bell pepper, cored,
   seeded, and cut into
   ½-inch-wide strips
1 green bell pepper, cored,
   seeded, and cut into
   ½-inch-wide strips
½ medium onion,
   thinly sliced
2 garlic cloves, minced
1 pound flank steak, cut
   into ½-inch-wide strips
Pink Himalayan sea salt
Freshly ground
   black pepper
¼ cup coconut aminos or
   soy sauce
2 tablespoons granulated
   erythritol
1 teaspoon ground ginger
Cauliflower rice, cooked
   (optional)

This Asian-inspired dish is a mix of tender bell peppers, onion, and flank steak served in a tangy ginger sauce. This is my go-to recipe when I want to order takeout but don't want to get off track with my diet. I typically serve this with cauliflower rice, but it's a fantastic meal on its own.

1. In a large sauté pan or skillet, heat 1 tablespoon of olive oil over medium heat. Add the bell peppers, onion, and garlic and cook until tender, about 5 minutes. Transfer the vegetables to a bowl.

2. Season the steak with salt and pepper and transfer it to the skillet. If there is no oil left in the pan, add about 1 teaspoon olive oil.

3. Increase the temperature to medium high and cook the steak for 5 to 7 minutes, with 5 minutes being for medium and 7 minutes being for well done.

4. In a small bowl, mix the coconut aminos, erythritol, and ginger.

5. Return the pepper mixture to the pan and drizzle with the sauce.

6. Reduce the heat to medium low and simmer for about 5 minutes, until the sauce reduces by about half, then serve with the cauliflower rice, if desired.

Macronutrients: 44% Fat, 46% Protein, 9% Carbs

Per serving: Calories: 316; Total Fat: 16g; Protein: 35g; Total Carbohydrates: 8g; Fiber: 2g; Erythritol: 12g; Net Carbs: 6g

Cheese-Stuffed Italian Meatballs

NUT FREE

Serves 4
Prep Time: 10 minutes
Cook Time: 30 minutes

For the meatballs

1 pound ground
   beef (80/20)
½ cup grated
   Parmesan cheese
1 large egg
2 teaspoons dried Italian
   seasoning
½ teaspoon pink Himalayan
   sea salt
½ teaspoon freshly ground
   black pepper
1 cup shredded
   low-moisture
   mozzarella cheese
Extra-virgin olive oil, for
   greasing

Ingredient List Continues ▸

If you've never had a meatball the size of your fist, stuffed with gooey mozzarella and smothered with marinara sauce, now's the time. These meatballs are full of the flavors of Italian herbs and Parmesan cheese. The molten cheese core provides melted mozzarella in every bite.

1. Preheat the oven to 350°F.

2. **To make the meatballs:** In a large bowl, combine the ground beef, Parmesan, egg, Italian seasoning, salt, and pepper. Using your hands, mix the meat the ingredients until well blended.

3. Divide the meat mixture into 4 equal portions, about 5 ounces each.

4. Flatten each portion into a square and fill the center of each with ¼ cup of the mozzarella. Fold the meat up and around the cheese to seal it well.

5. Coat an 8-inch square baking dish with some olive oil. Place the meatballs in the dish and bake for 30 minutes.

CONTINUES ▸

For the sauce

1 cup tomato puree

1 garlic clove, minced

½ teaspoon pink Himalayan
sea salt

½ teaspoon Italian
seasoning

6. **To make the sauce:** In a medium bowl, mix the tomato puree, garlic, salt, and Italian seasoning.

7. Top the meatballs in the baking pan with the sauce, then bake for an additional 8 to 10 minutes, until the sauce is heated through and coating the meatballs. Serve.

Storage Tip: This recipe makes 4 servings, so you'll probably want to save some leftovers. Store the meatballs in an airtight container in your refrigerator for 4 to 5 days. Make sure the meatballs are heated to the cheese core when you next serve them.

Macronutrients: 64% Fat, 28% Protein, 8% Carbs

Per serving: Calories: 478; Total Fat: 34g; Protein: 32g; Total Carbohydrates: 9g; Fiber: 1g; Erythritol: 0g; Net Carbs: 8g

Lamb and Beef Kebabs

NUT FREE

Serves 2
Prep Time: 15 Minutes
Cook Time: 25 Minutes

Coconut oil cooking spray
¼ medium onion, chopped
8 ounces ground
    beef (80/20)
8 ounces ground lamb
1 large egg
1 garlic clove, minced
½ teaspoon pink Himalayan
    sea salt
½ teaspoon freshly ground
    black pepper
½ teaspoon ground sumac
¼ teaspoon ground
    turmeric
2 tablespoons
    butter, melted

This recipe was inspired by the many different Middle Eastern restaurants I've eaten in over the years. There's something wonderful about the blend of beef, lamb, and spices of the region. These kebabs are incredibly juicy, filled with the flavors of sumac and turmeric. They will also definitely boost your fat macronutrients for the day.

1. Preheat the oven to 450°F. Line a large baking sheet with aluminum foil and spray with the cooking spray.

2. In a food processor, puree the onion on high speed until a smooth paste forms. You may need to scrape down the sides of the bowl.

3. Transfer the onion paste to a fine-mesh strainer over the sink and toss it around a few times to drain off any liquid.

4. In a large bowl, combine the onion paste with the beef, lamb, egg, garlic, salt, pepper, sumac, and turmeric. Using your hands, mix the meat with the seasonings until well combined.

5. Divide the mixture into 4 equal portions, then roll each into a cylinder. Slide metal skewers through the cylinders, if desired, or you can bake them as is.

6. Transfer the kebabs to the baking sheet and bake for 15 minutes.

CONTINUES ▶

7. Brush the tops of the kebabs with the melted butter, then return them to the oven for an additional 5 to 10 minutes of baking. An instant-read thermometer should reach 155°F when inserted in the center, and no pink should remain in the meat.

8. Let the kebabs cool for 5 minutes, then serve.

> **Ingredient Tip:** Ground lamb can, on occasion, be expensive or hard to find. The same goes for sumac. If you can't use lamb, double the amount of beef. If you need a sumac substitute, try ¼ teaspoon lemon zest and ¼ teaspoon ground black pepper—though I recommend trying to find both of these tasty ingredients, if you can.

Macronutrients: 75% Fat, 24% Protein, 1% Carbs

Per serving: Calories: 724; Total Fat: 60g; Protein: 46g; Total Carbohydrates: 2g; Fiber: 0g; Erythritol: 0g; Net Carbs: 2g

Pork Larb Lettuce Wraps

DAIRY FREE, EGG FREE, NUT FREE, UNDER 30 MINUTES

Serves 2
Prep Time: 8 minutes
Cook Time: 20 minutes

1 pound ground pork
¼ medium onion,
  finely chopped
1 fresh long red chile,
  thinly sliced
2 garlic cloves, minced
Juice of 1 lime
2 tablespoons chopped
  fresh basil
1 tablespoon chopped
  fresh cilantro or dried
  coriander
1 tablespoon fish sauce
1 teaspoon granulated
  erythritol
1 teaspoon dried mint
1 tablespoon extra-virgin
  olive oil
Pink Himalayan sea salt
Freshly ground
  black pepper
4 large, firm leaves
  of iceberg or
  butterhead lettuce
4 lime wedges, for garnish

Larb is a bright and fresh meat salad from the areas surrounding Laos and Thailand. It uses a variety of herbs to create a unique flavor, but fresh basil is the most notable. The sauce is a little bit salty and acidic, but full of fresh citrus flavor. The larb is then served in a crisp lettuce wrap to lend a nice crunch to the dish.

1. In a large bowl, combine the pork, onion, chile, and garlic.

2. In a small bowl, combine the lime juice, basil, cilantro, fish sauce, erythritol, and mint.

3. In a large sauté pan or skillet, heat the olive oil over medium-high heat. Add the pork mixture and cook for 8 to 10 minutes, until no pink remains.

4. Add the sauce and cook for 5 to 8 minutes more, until most of the sauce is reduced. Season with salt and pepper.

5. Divide the meat mixture among the 4 lettuce leaves, fold into wraps, and serve with a wedge of lime.

Ingredient Tip: Thai or Vietnamese fish sauce often contains hidden sugars. Verify that the fish sauce you are using does not contain any sugars.

Macronutrients: 73% Fat, 25% Protein, 2% Carbs

Per serving: Calories: 675; Total Fat: 55g; Protein: 39g; Total Carbohydrates: 5g; Fiber: 0g; Erythritol: 2g; Net Carbs: 5g

Smothered Pork Chops

EGG FREE, NUT FREE, ONE PAN

Serves 2
Prep Time: 5 minutes
Cook Time: 35 minutes

1 tablespoon extra-virgin
  olive oil
2 large loin pork chops
¼ teaspoon ground sage
Pink Himalayan sea salt
Freshly ground
  black pepper
½ medium onion, sliced
1 tablespoon butter
2 garlic cloves, minced
½ cup chicken broth
¼ cup heavy
  (whipping) cream

These pork chops are smothered with onions and a creamy gravy—possibly the best way to enjoy pork. The gravy is my favorite part of this dish, as it lends a slightly salty richness, while the caramelized onion graces the dish with a bit of sweetness.

1. In a medium sauté pan or skillet, heat the olive oil over medium-high heat.

2. Season the pork chops with the sage, salt, and pepper.

3. Add the chops to the hot oil and cook for about 5 minutes per side; the chops should be golden brown. Transfer the chops to a plate.

4. Reduce the heat to medium low and add the onion and butter to the skillet. Cook for 12 to 15 minutes, stirring occasionally, until caramelized.

5. Add the garlic and cook for 1 more minute. Add the broth, then add the cream. Stir slowly, until the sauce starts to simmer.

6. Return the pork chops and any juices to the skillet. Simmer for about 10 minutes, until the chops are cooked through and the sauce has thickened.

7. Season with salt and pepper, then serve immediately.

Variation Tip: Seasoning the pork with poultry seasoning instead of the sage creates a slightly different flavor profile, should you be looking to vary this a bit.

Macronutrients: 65% Fat, 32% Protein, 3% Carbs

Per serving: Calories: 567; Total Fat: 41g; Protein: 42g; Total Carbohydrates: 4g; Fiber: 1g; Erythritol: 0g; Net Carbs: 3g

Fried Rice with Ham

NUT FREE, ONE PAN, UNDER 30 MINUTES

Serves 2
Prep Time: 5 minutes
Cook Time: 20 minutes

2 tablespoons butter

12 ounces boneless cooked
ham steak, cubed

¼ medium onion, chopped

1 teaspoon minced garlic

1 (12-ounce) package
cauliflower rice, fresh or
thawed frozen

¼ cup peas, fresh or
thawed frozen

2 tablespoons coconut
aminos or soy sauce

½ teaspoon rice
wine vinegar

¼ teaspoon pink Himalayan
sea salt

¼ teaspoon freshly ground
black pepper

1 tablespoon extra-virgin
olive oil

2 large eggs

A few years ago, I wanted to make fried cauliflower rice for dinner but couldn't find a good protein to add to it. I had some ham steak in the refrigerator from the night before, and I decided to try it. Boy, am I glad I did! This dish has become a staple in my house, spiking the cauliflower with the juicy, salty flavors of ham.

1. In a large sauté pan or skillet, melt the butter over medium heat. Add the ham cubes and cook for about 5 minutes, stirring, until slightly crisp on all sides.

2. Add the onion and cook for 3 to 5 minutes, until translucent. Then add the garlic and cook for an additional minute, until fragrant.

3. Mix the cauliflower rice and peas into the skillet and cook for 3 to 5 minutes, stirring from time to time.

4. In a small bowl, combine the coconut aminos, vinegar, salt, and pepper.

5. Add the sauce mixture to the pan and stir to coat well. Continue to stir and cook until the cauliflower rice and peas are warmed through.

6. Push the mixture to one side of the skillet, then add the olive oil to the other side. Heat the oil for 30 seconds to 1 minute, then add the eggs. Using a spatula or wooden spoon, scramble the eggs for 2 to 3 minutes, until cooked.

CONTINUES ▶

7. Stir the cauliflower mixture into the eggs, combining all ingredients in the skillet, until slightly browned and heated through. Serve.

Variation Tip: You can use just about any other protein for this recipe or you can completely leave it out to make this a vegetarian dish. If you don't mind some of the ingredients in Spam, its carb count is low enough to make this a Spam fried rice.

Macronutrients: 56% Fat, 36% Protein, 8% Carbs

Per serving: Calories: 536; Total Fat: 32g; Protein: 46g; Total Carbohydrates: 17g; Fiber: 7g; Erythritol: 0g; Net Carbs: 10g

Crispy Bourbon Pork Belly

DAIRY FREE, EGG FREE, NUT FREE

Serves 4
Prep Time: 10 minutes
Cook Time: 3 hours

In this decadent recipe, pork belly is slow-cooked in Kentucky bourbon, then crisped on all sides and coated with a sweet and smoky sauce.

For the pork belly

1 pound pork belly, skin
  removed, cut into
  1-inch cubes
Pink Himalayan sea salt
Freshly ground
  black pepper
1½ ounces (3 tablespoons)
  Kentucky bourbon

For the sauce

1½ ounces (3 tablespoons)
  Kentucky bourbon
2 tablespoons
  sugar-free ketchup
1 tablespoon granulated
  erythritol
2 teaspoons
  coconut aminos
¼ teaspoon freshly ground
  black pepper
Dash of liquid smoke
Pinch of Pink Himalayan
  sea salt

1. Preheat the oven to 300°F.

2. **To make the pork belly:** Season the pork belly with salt and pepper. Place the pork in an 8-inch baking pan and pour over the bourbon. Cover the pan tightly with aluminum foil and bake for 2 hours and 30 minutes.

3. Remove the foil and drain the juices from the pan.

4. Turn the oven up to 425°F and bake the pork for 20 minutes more, until crispy. If it's not crisp enough for your liking, place it under the broiler for a few minutes.

5. **To make the sauce:** In a small saucepan over medium heat, combine the bourbon, ketchup, erythritol, coconut aminos, pepper, liquid smoke, and salt. Simmer for 5 to 7 minutes, stirring occasionally, until the sauce reduces by half.

6. Add the sauce to the pork in the pan and turn the meat to coat with the sauce.

7. Bake for an additional 5 minutes, then serve.

Ingredient Tip: Removing the skin from pork belly can be fairly challenging. If possible, buy the pork belly with the skin already removed. Your butcher should be able to do this for you.

Macronutrients: 92% Fat, 8% Protein, 0% Carbs

Per serving: Calories: 638; Total Fat: 60g; Protein: 11g; Total Carbohydrates: 0g; Fiber: 0g; Erythritol: 8g; Net Carbs: 0g

Spicy Barbecued Pork Wings

EGG FREE, NUT FREE

Serves 2
Prep Time: 10 minutes
Cook Time: 10 minutes to
3 hours

4 pork wings or trimmed
   pork shanks
¼ cup water
1 teaspoon extra-virgin
   olive oil
¼ cup sugar-free
   barbecue sauce
2 tablespoons butter
1 teaspoon hot sauce
   of choice
Cayenne pepper

If pigs could fly, I bet their wings would be delicious. But since they can't, this is the next best thing. The "wings" are actually part of the shank that has been trimmed to look like a drumstick. Most butchers sell them as "pig wings" or "pork wings," and often they are already cooked. These wings are then crisped and covered in a spicy barbecue sauce. Don't wait until pigs actually fly to try this recipe!

1. If the wings did not come already cooked, preheat the oven to 300°F. (If they did, skip to step 3.)

2. Place the wings in an 8-inch square baking pan and add the water. Seal the pan with aluminum foil. Bake for 2 to 3 hours, until the meat is tender.

3. In a medium sauté pan or skillet, heat the olive oil over medium-high heat. Add the wings and crisp for 2 to 3 minutes on each side.

4. Transfer the pork to a platter. Lower the heat to medium and add the barbecue sauce, butter, and hot sauce to the skillet. Season to taste with cayenne.

5. Stir the sauce until it starts to simmer, then put the wings back in the skillet and coat with the sauce.

6. Simmer until the sauce has thickened and sticks to the wings, about 2 minutes. Serve.

Macronutrients: 67% Fat, 32% Protein, 1% Carbs

Per serving: Calories: 458; Total Fat: 35g; Protein: 34g; Total Carbohydrates: 2g; Fiber: 1g; Erythritol: 6g; Net Carbs: 1g

Breaded Pork Chops

EGG FREE, NUT FREE, ONE PAN, UNDER 30 MINUTES

Serves 2
Prep Time: 5 minutes
Cook Time: 20 Minutes

2 (8-ounce) boneless pork
    loin chops
¼ cup pork panko crumbs
    (see Tip, page 60)
1 teaspoon extra-virgin
    olive oil
1 teaspoon grated
    Parmesan cheese
¼ teaspoon pink Himalayan
    sea salt
¼ teaspoon onion powder
¼ teaspoon paprika
¼ teaspoon garlic powder
⅛ teaspoon freshly ground
    black pepper
⅛ teaspoon dried parsley
⅛ teaspoon dried basil
⅛ teaspoon dried oregano
Pinch of cayenne pepper

If you're missing those flavored bread crumbs that turn an ordinary pork chop into a flavor-packed meal, here's your solution. This is an easy, well-seasoned, and keto-friendly breading for chops that clings to the meat and crisps up nicely to form that golden-brown coating we all know and love.

1. Preheat the oven to 425°F. Place a baking rack on a small baking sheet.

2. Pat the chops dry with a paper towel.

3. In a food processor, combine the pork crumbs, olive oil, Parmesan, salt, onion powder, paprika, garlic powder, pepper, parsley, basil, oregano, and cayenne and run on high until the mixture forms a uniform, fine powder. Transfer the mixture to a resealable 1-gallon plastic bag.

4. Add the chops to the bag, one at a time, shaking to coat them in the breading.

5. Transfer the chops to the rack and bake for 20 minutes, until an instant-read thermometer registers 160°F or the juices run clear when the meat is pierced.

Variation Tip: If you don't like pork chops or just want to change the protein, then substitute boneless, skinless chicken thighs for an equally great result.

Macronutrients: 48% Fat, 52% Protein, 0% Carbs

Per serving: Calories: 435; Total Fat: 23g; Protein: 57g; Total Carbohydrates: 0g; Fiber: 0g; Erythritol: 0g; Net Carbs: 0g

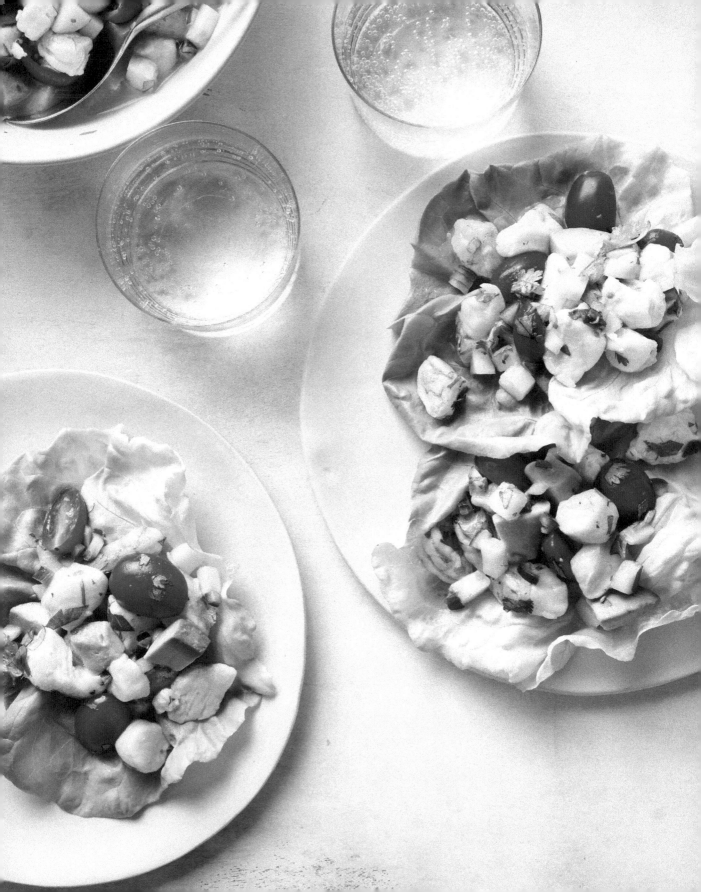

Fish and Seafood

Parmesan-Crusted Salmon

EGG FREE, NUT FREE, UNDER 30 MINUTES

Serves 2
Prep Time: 5 minutes
Cook Time: 20 minutes

2 tablespoons mayonnaise

1 tablespoon grated
Parmesan cheese

1 tablespoon shredded
Parmesan cheese

1 teaspoon freshly
squeezed lemon juice

½ teaspoon dried parsley

½ teaspoon minced garlic

Pink Himalayan sea salt

Freshly ground
black pepper

2 (8-ounce) salmon
fillets, skin on

This salmon dish provides all the fats you need on a keto diet. The fish is juicy and flaky but holds together well, topped with a sauce full of the flavors of Parmesan cheese, lemon, garlic, and parsley.

1. Preheat the oven to 400°F. Line a baking sheet with aluminum foil.

2. In a small bowl, combine the mayonnaise, both types of Parmesan, lemon juice, parsley, and garlic. Season with salt and pepper.

3. Place the salmon skin-side down on the baking sheet. Spread the sauce evenly across both fillets.

4. Bake for 15 to 17 minutes, until the salmon flakes easily with a fork. Serve immediately.

Cooking Tip: Because the foil on the baking sheet is not greased, the skin of the fish sticks to it and makes it easier to remove just the meat. Slide a flat spatula between the skin and the meat to pull the fish off cleanly.

Macronutrients: 62% Fat, 37% Protein, 1% Carbs

Per serving: Calories: 584; Total Fat: 40g; Protein: 53g; Total Carbohydrates: 1g; Fiber: 0g; Erythritol: 0g; Net Carbs: 1g

Cod Cakes

DAIRY FREE, UNDER 30 MINUTES

Serves 2
Prep Time: 5 minutes
Cook Time: 20 minutes

2 tablespoons plus
  1 teaspoon extra-virgin
  olive oil, divided
¼ medium onion, chopped
1 garlic clove, minced
1 cup cauliflower rice, fresh
  or thawed frozen
1 pound cod fillets
½ cup almond flour
1 large egg
2 tablespoons chopped
  fresh parsley
2 tablespoons ground
  flaxseed
1 tablespoon freshly
  squeezed lemon juice
1 teaspoon dried dill
½ teaspoon ground cumin
½ teaspoon pink Himalayan
  sea salt
¼ teaspoon freshly ground
  black pepper
Tartar sauce

I have always loved a good crab or fish cake, and these are no exception. This preparation uses cod, but just about any other white fish will work as well. These are crispy and don't skimp on flavor, complemented by the slightly smoky taste of cumin and the hint of dill. If you love a good fish cake and want to keep keto, give these a try!

1. In a medium sauté pan or skillet, heat 1 tablespoon of olive oil over medium heat. Add the onion and garlic and cook for about 7 minutes, until tender.

2. Add the cauliflower rice and continue to stir for 5 to 7 minutes, until warmed through and tender. Transfer to a large bowl.

3. In the same skillet, heat 1 teaspoon of olive oil over medium-high heat. Cook the cod for 4 to 5 minutes on each side, until cooked through. Let the cod cool for a couple of minutes.

4. Add the almond flour, egg, parsley, flaxseed, lemon juice, dill, cumin, salt, and pepper to the bowl with the cauliflower rice. Using your hands, mix until the ingredients are well combined.

5. Add the fish to the bowl and mix well. I like to use a fluffing motion to keep the fish in chunks, rather than smashing it all.

6. In the skillet, heat the remaining 1 tablespoon of olive oil over medium heat.

CONTINUES ▶

7. Using a ½ cup measuring cup, form the fish cakes by packing the mixture into the cup, then slipping the cake out of the cup onto a plate. You should be able to shape 4 cakes.

8. Place the fish cakes in the hot oil and cook for about 5 minutes per side, flipping once, until golden brown on both sides.

9. Place the cod cakes on serving plates, and serve with tartar sauce.

Variation Tip: This recipe makes wonderful crab cakes as well. Use 1 pound of lump crab meat, and you'll have yourself delicious crab cakes.

Macronutrients: 56% Fat, 35% Protein, 9% Carbs

Per serving: Calories: 531; Total Fat: 34g; Protein: 45g; Total Carbohydrates: 12g; Fiber: 6g; Erythritol: 0g; Net Carbs: 6g

Tuna Salad Wrap

NUT FREE, ONE BOWL, UNDER 30 MINUTES

Serves 2

Prep Time: 5 minutes

2 (5-ounce) cans tuna packed in olive oil, drained (see Tip)

3 tablespoons mayonnaise

1 tablespoon chopped red onion

2 teaspoons dill relish

¼ teaspoon pink Himalayan sea salt

¼ teaspoon freshly ground black pepper

Pinch of dried or fresh dill

2 low-carb tortillas

2 romaine lettuce leaves

¼ cup grated cheddar cheese

A classic tuna salad wrap is a simple and flavorful meal that can be ready in around five minutes. A low-carb tortilla, whether store-bought or homemade, provides the sturdy edible holder for crisp romaine lettuce, a bit of sharp cheddar cheese, and of course the tuna salad. The salad itself provides plenty of healthy fats and is loaded with the flavors of dill, onion, and a hint of black pepper. Whether it's for a weekday lunch or a quick and easy dinner, this is one to enjoy again and again.

1. In a medium bowl, combine the tuna, mayonnaise, onion, relish, salt, pepper, and dill.

2. Place a lettuce leaf on each tortilla, then split the tuna mixture evenly between the wraps, spreading it evenly over the lettuce.

3. Sprinkle the cheddar on top of each, then fold the tortillas and serve.

Ingredient Tip: Sometimes tuna comes packed in oils other than olive oil. These oils will not have an impact on ketosis, but they aren't necessarily great for your body. If you can find it, use tuna in olive oil. If not, tuna packed in water is a good option.

Macronutrients: 54% Fat, 31% Protein, 15% Carbs

Per serving: Calories: 549; Total Fat: 33g; Protein: 42g; Total Carbohydrates: 21g; Fiber: 16g; Erythritol: 0g; Net Carbs: 5g

Pan-Seared Lemon-Garlic Salmon

EGG FREE, NUT FREE, ONE PAN, UNDER 30 MINUTES

Serves 2
Prep Time: 5 minutes
Cook Time: 10 minutes

1 tablespoon extra-virgin
   olive oil
2 (8-ounce) salmon fillets
1 lemon, halved
Pink Himalayan sea salt
Freshly ground
   black pepper
2 tablespoons butter
1 tablespoon chopped
   fresh parsley
2 garlic cloves, minced

This dish allows the salmon to be the star of the show, instead of hiding it under other strong flavors. The salmon fillet is simply seasoned with lemon juice, salt, and pepper, then pan-seared to add a slight crust. The natural flavors of the fish are enhanced with the tartness of the lemon juice and a hint of garlic. The buttery sauce helps keep your fats on track for a keto diet.

1. In a medium sauté pan or skillet, heat the olive oil over medium-high heat.

2. Squeeze the juice from a lemon half over the fillets. Season the salmon with salt and pepper.

3. Place the salmon skin-side up in the skillet. Cook for 4 to 5 minutes, then flip the fish and cook for an additional 2 to 3 minutes on the other side.

4. Add the butter, the juice from the other lemon half, the parsley, and garlic to the pan. Toss to combine. Allow the fish to cook for 2 to 3 more minutes, until the flesh flakes easily with a fork.

5. Transfer the fish to a serving plate, then top with the butter sauce and serve.

Macronutrients: 60% Fat, 39% Protein, 1% Carbs

Per serving: Calories: 489; Total Fat: 33g; Protein: 45g; Total Carbohydrates: 0g; Fiber: 0g; Erythritol: 0g; Net Carbs: 1g

Coconut Shrimp

DAIRY FREE

Serves 2
Prep Time: 10 minutes
Cook Time: 25 minutes

Coconut oil cooking spray
12 extra-jumbo shrimp, peeled, tails on
3 tablespoons coconut flour
1 tablespoon granulated erythritol
½ teaspoon pink Himalayan sea salt
¼ teaspoon baking powder
¼ teaspoon freshly ground black pepper
2 large eggs
¼ cup soda water
½ cup unsweetened shredded coconut
½ cup pork panko crumbs (see Tip)

These crispy coconut shrimp can compete with the best of them. The exterior coating gives a satisfying crunch with every bite. The batter is made with coconut flour, to emphasize the taste of coconut, while the pork panko and coconut-flake coating makes it look and feel like its non-keto counterpart.

1. Preheat the oven to 425°F. Line an 8-inch square baking pan with aluminum foil and spray with the cooking spray.

2. Pat the shrimp dry, then place in a medium bowl. Add 1 tablespoon of the coconut flour and toss to coat the shrimp.

3. In a small bowl, combine the remaining 2 tablespoons coconut flour, the erythritol, salt, baking powder, and pepper. Mix with a whisk to break up any clumps.

4. Create a well in the center of the dry ingredients, then add the eggs and the soda water to the well. Scramble the eggs into the soda water, then start to stir in the dry ingredients until a thin batter forms.

5. On a large plate, combine the shredded coconut and pork crumbs.

6. Place the bowls of shrimp, batter, and coating in a line on the counter.

7. Take a shrimp, dip it in the batter, shake off the excess batter, then toss in the coconut coating. Place the shrimp in the baking pan, and repeat for the remaining shrimp.

CONTINUES ▶

8. Spray the tops of the shrimp with the cooking spray. This helps to crisp the shrimp.

9. Bake for 15 to 17 minutes. Then, set the broiler on high and broil for 3 to 5 minutes, until the coating is golden brown and crispy. Serve.

Ingredient Tip: Pork panko crumbs are available at most Asian markets, but they can also be easily made at home by processing a bag of unflavored pork rinds in a food processor until you have fine crumbs.

Variation Tip: If you enjoy the flavor of a beer batter, swap out the soda water for your favorite low-carb beer.

Macronutrients: 60% Fat, 34% Protein, 6% Carbs

Per serving: Calories: 349; Total Fat: 23g; Protein: 30g; Total Carbohydrates: 7g; Fiber: 4g; Erythritol: 6g; Net Carbs: 3g

Bacon-Wrapped Shrimp

DAIRY FREE, EGG FREE, NUT FREE, UNDER 30 MINUTES

Serves 2
Prep Time: 5 minutes
Cook Time: 20 minutes

1 teaspoon granulated
   erythritol
½ teaspoon chili powder
¼ teaspoon pink Himalayan
   sea salt
¼ teaspoon freshly ground
   black pepper
¼ teaspoon onion powder
12 extra-jumbo shrimp,
   peeled, tails on
6 slices bacon

What is better than seafood and bacon? How about seafood wrapped in bacon? This dish is quickly becoming a favorite in my house. The crispy, salty bacon is the perfect mate for the softer, slightly sweet shrimp. The shrimp are seasoned with a pinch of onion and chili powder to tie it all together.

1. Preheat the oven to 400°F. Line a baking sheet with aluminum foil.

2. In a small bowl, combine the erythritol, chili powder, salt, pepper, and onion powder.

3. In a medium bowl, combine the shrimp with the spice mixture, tossing the shrimp around to evenly distribute the seasoning.

4. Cut the bacon strips in half crosswise. Wrap each shrimp with one of the pieces, using the slight overlap to hold it together. Place the bacon-wrapped shrimp on the baking sheet with the loose ends of bacon on the undersides.

5. Bake for 18 to 20 minutes, until the bacon is crisp.

6. Allow the shrimp to cool for about 5 minutes, then serve.

Variation Tip: To add a nice sauce to this shrimp dish, drizzle with a keto-friendly barbecue sauce during the last 5 minutes of cooking.

Macronutrients: 60% Fat, 37% Protein, 3% Carbs

Per serving: Calories: 194; Total Fat: 13g; Protein: 17g; Total Carbohydrates: 2g; Fiber: 0g; Erythritol: 2g; Net Carbs: 2g

Crab au Gratin

EGG FREE, NUT FREE

Serves 4
Prep Time: 10 minutes
Cook Time: 35 minutes

This recipe turns a classic crab au gratin into a rich casserole. Instead of serving it with a side of chips or crostini, our keto variation mixes cauliflower rice right into the dish.

½ cup (1 stick) butter

1 (8-ounce) container crab claw meat

2 ounces full-fat cream cheese

½ cup heavy (whipping) cream

2 tablespoons freshly squeezed lemon juice

1 tablespoon white wine vinegar

1 teaspoon pink Himalayan sea salt

½ teaspoon freshly ground black pepper

½ teaspoon onion powder

1 cup shredded cheddar cheese, divided

1 (12-ounce) package cauliflower rice, cooked and drained

1. Preheat the oven to 350°F.

2. In a medium sauté pan or skillet, melt the butter over medium heat. Add the crab and cook until warmed through.

3. Add the cream cheese, cream, lemon juice, vinegar, salt, pepper, and onion powder. Keep stirring until the cream cheese fully melts into the sauce.

4. Add ½ cup of cheddar cheese and stir it into the sauce.

5. Spread the cauliflower rice on the bottom of an 8-inch square baking dish.

6. Pour the crab and sauce over, then sprinkle with the remaining ½ cup of cheddar cheese.

7. Bake for 25 to 30 minutes, until the sauce is bubbling. Turn the broiler on to high.

8. Broil for an additional 2 to 3 minutes, until the cheese topping is slightly browned.

9. Allow to cool for 5 to 10 minutes, then serve.

Ingredient Tip: It may be tempting to buy imitation crab, but don't. It is typically loaded with carbs from all the fillers, and it is not much cheaper than claw meat, which is less expensive than lump.

Macronutrients: 79% Fat, 17% Protein, 4% Carbs

Per serving: Calories: 555; Total Fat: 49g; Protein: 23g; Total Carbohydrates: 7g; Fiber: 2g; Erythritol: 0g; Net Carbs: 5g

Salmon Oscar

NUT FREE, UNDER 30 MINUTES

Serves 2
Prep Time: 5 minutes
Cook Time: 20 minutes

¼ cup (½ stick) butter
1 tablespoon finely
   minced onion
1½ teaspoons white
   wine vinegar
1 teaspoon freshly
   squeezed lemon juice
½ teaspoon dried tarragon
¼ teaspoon dried parsley
1 large egg yolk
2 tablespoons heavy
   (whipping) cream
1 tablespoon extra-virgin
   olive oil
2 (8-ounce) salmon fillets
Pink Himalayan sea salt
Freshly ground
   black pepper
1 (6- to 8-ounce) container
   lump crab meat

Cooking salmon Oscar style adds flavor and fat to an otherwise simple fillet of fish. In this case, the salmon is graced with a generous portion of lump crab meat and a homemade bearnaise sauce. Don't let the fancy sauce intimidate you—it's easy to make and packs a ton of flavor.

1. In a small saucepan, melt the butter over medium heat.

2. Add the onion and cook for 3 to 5 minutes, until it begins to turn translucent. Add the vinegar, lemon juice, tarragon, and parsley. Stir to combine.

3. In a small bowl, whisk together the egg yolk and cream.

4. Once the mixture in the saucepan starts to simmer, remove it from the heat and slowly add the egg mixture, whisking while you pour. Continue to whisk for 2 to 3 minutes, until the sauce thickens. Cover and set aside.

5. Season the salmon fillets with salt and pepper.

6. In a medium sauté pan or skillet, heat the olive oil over medium-high heat. Place the fillets skin-side up in the skillet. Cook for 4 to 5 minutes, then turn and cook for an additional 4 to 5 minutes on the other side, until the flesh flakes easily with a fork.

CONTINUES ▶

7. Transfer the salmon to a serving plate, then place the crab in the skillet and quickly heat it, stirring gently.

8. Top the salmon fillets with the crab, then drizzle on the sauce. Serve at once.

Cooking Tip: If the sauce comes to a boil, it will separate. If that happens, add a splash of cream and whisk vigorously until it recombines.

Macronutrients: 63% Fat, 36% Protein, 1% Carbs

Per serving: Calories: 741; Total Fat: 53g; Protein: 62g; Total Carbohydrates: 1g; Fiber: 0g; Erythritol: 0g; Net Carbs: 1g

Garlic-Butter Scallops

EGG FREE, NUT FREE, ONE PAN, UNDER 15 MINUTES

Serves 2
Prep Time: 2 minutes
Cook Time: 10 minutes

1 tablespoon extra-virgin
olive oil
8 firm sea scallops (about
8 ounces)
Pink Himalayan sea salt
Freshly ground
black pepper
3 tablespoons butter
1 garlic clove, minced

When preparing scallops, I often find that less is more—that is, simple preparations allow the scallop flavor to shine. Here, the scallops are seasoned with salt and pepper, then pan-seared to gain a crunchy crust. They are finished with melted butter and garlic, adding a little bit of flavor and fat. The simplicity of this dish makes it a great option for a quick meal.

1. In a medium sauté pan or skillet, heat the olive oil over medium heat.

2. Season the scallops with salt and pepper, then place in the skillet and cook for 5 minutes.

3. Carefully turn the scallops and cook for an additional 3 minutes on the other side. The scallops will form a nice crust.

4. Add the butter and garlic to the skillet. Allow the butter to melt and the garlic to become aromatic, just a few minutes.

5. Transfer the scallops to a serving plate, and pour the seasoned butter over the top.

Macronutrients: 74% Fat, 20% Protein, 6% Carbs

Per serving: Calories: 293; Total Fat: 25g; Protein: 14g; Total Carbohydrates: 4g; Fiber: 0g; Erythritol: 0g; Net Carbs: 4g

Fish and Scallop Ceviche

DAIRY FREE, EGG FREE, NUT FREE, ONE BOWL

Serves 3

Prep Time: 10 minutes,
plus 1 hour to chill

4 ounces shrimp, peeled
and chopped

1 (4-ounce) white fish
fillet, chopped into
bite-size pieces

4 ounces bay or other
small scallops

¼ small red onion, chopped

½ jalapeño pepper, seeded
and finely chopped

1 garlic clove, minced

½ teaspoon pink Himalayan
sea salt

¼ teaspoon freshly ground
black pepper

3 or 4 limes

½ medium cucumber,
peeled and chopped

½ avocado, slightly
firm, chopped

⅓ cup grape
tomatoes, halved

3 tablespoons chopped
fresh cilantro

2 teaspoons extra-virgin
olive oil

Firm lettuce leaves,
for wraps

Whether you serve ceviche in a lettuce wrap or as is, you won't find an easier summer meal. The flavors are both fresh and bright, thanks to the lime juice used to "cook" the raw fish. Avocado is added for its nutrients and healthy fats. I like to use red snapper, but any white fish will work for this delicious dish.

1. In a large bowl, combine the shrimp, fish, and scallops.

2. Add the red onion, jalapeño, garlic, salt, and pepper. Using a wooden spoon, stir to mix the ingredients.

3. Roll the limes on the countertop, pressing firmly down with your hand to soften. Slice the limes in half crosswise, then squeeze the juice into the bowl and stir well.

4. Cover the bowl with plastic wrap, and place in the refrigerator for 45 minutes to 1 hour.

5. Add the cucumber, avocado, tomatoes, and cilantro to the bowl. Gently mix, trying not to smash the avocado.

6. Drizzle the ceviche with the olive oil, then serve with the lettuce to make wraps.

> **Ingredient Tip**: Ultra-fresh ingredients are key when it comes to ceviche. The acidity of the lime does "cook" the fish, but the fresh taste is much better if you start with great ingredients.

Macronutrients: 38% Fat, 41% Protein, 21% Carbs

Per serving: Calories: 211; Total Fat: 9g; Protein: 21g; Total Carbohydrates: 13g; Fiber: 4g; Erythritol: 0g; Net Carbs: 9g

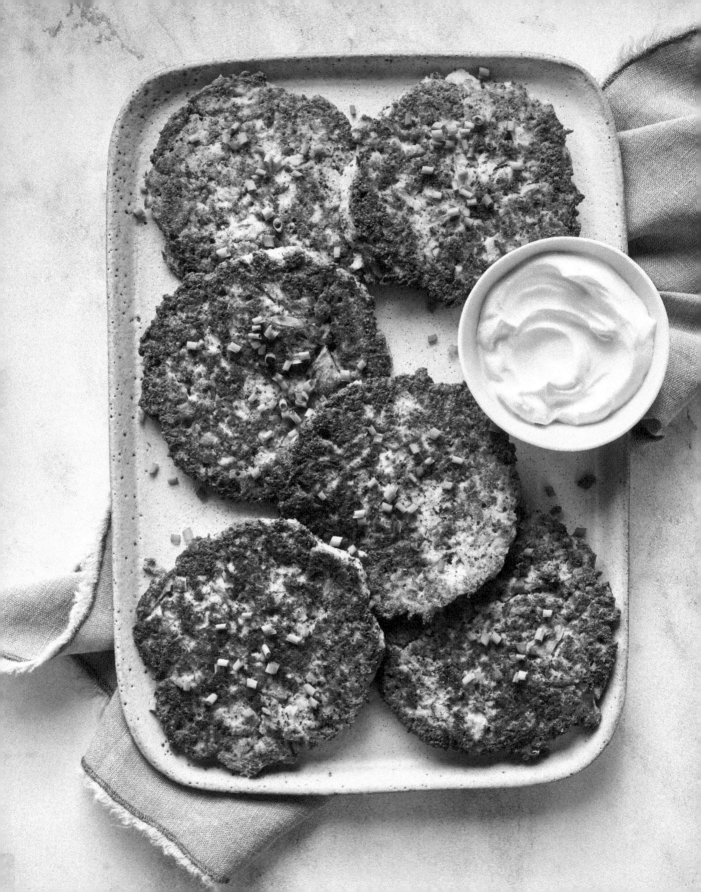

CHAPTER EIGHT

Vegetable Sides and Mains

Bacon Green Beans

DAIRY FREE, EGG FREE, NUT FREE, ONE PAN, UNDER 30 MINUTES

Serves 2
Prep Time: 2 minutes
Cook Time: 20 minutes

2 ounces (2 to 3 strips)
   bacon, cut into ½-inch-
   wide crosswise strips
6 ounces green
   beans, trimmed
½ teaspoon seasoning salt
¼ teaspoon red
   pepper flakes

These green beans are perfect for those days when you don't really want to make a side dish, but you know you need some vegetables. The bacon adds crunch and provides the fat for cooking the beans. Add the seasoning salt and red pepper to it and you're good to go.

1. Heat a medium sauté pan or skillet over medium-high heat, then add the bacon. Cook for 7 to 10 minutes, until the bacon is almost crispy.

2. Reduce the heat to medium low and add the beans, seasoning salt, and red pepper flakes.

3. Sauté the beans for 7 to 10 minutes, until tender but still crisp.

4. Transfer to a serving plate and enjoy!

Variation Tip: This same technique works great with halved or whole Brussels sprouts. They take a bit longer to cook, so add them just before the bacon is done cooking.

Serving Tip: These green beans go great with the Braised Short Ribs (page 77). After indulging in the rich and tender short rib, these crisp and fresh green beans offer a great counterbalance.

Macronutrients: 72% Fat, 13% Protein, 15% Carbs

Per serving: Calories: 142; Total Fat: 11g; Protein: 5g; Total Carbohydrates: 6g; Fiber: 2g; Erythritol: 0g; Net Carbs: 4g

Mashed Cauliflower

EGG FREE, NUT FREE, UNDER 20 MINUTES, VEGETARIAN

Serves 2
Prep Time: 10 minutes
Cook Time: 10 minutes

8 ounces cauliflower
   florets, fresh or frozen
   (about 2 cups)
2 tablespoons water
2 ounces full-fat
   cream cheese
2 tablespoons butter
½ teaspoon pink Himalayan
   sea salt
¼ teaspoon freshly ground
   black pepper

Mashed cauliflower is a side dish I first made when I had just started a keto diet. The texture and taste of the pureed cauliflower is incredibly similar to mashed potatoes, but this dish has a carb count that is perfect for this diet. Season the mash with some salt and butter, and you'll have those mashed potatoes you were missing.

1. Add the cauliflower to a medium microwave-safe bowl along with the water, and microwave on high power for 6 to 8 minutes. (Alternatively, you can steam the cauliflower until very tender.)

2. Drain the cauliflower—this is critical.

3. Transfer the cauliflower to a food processor and pulse to break the florets into much smaller pieces.

4. Add the cream cheese, butter, salt, and pepper. Process on high power until the cauliflower mash reaches your desired consistency. You may need to scrape down the sides of the bowl a few times using a rubber scraper. Serve immediately.

Variation Tip: To create a garlic and cheddar mash, simply add ¼ teaspoon garlic powder and ¼ cup grated cheddar cheese to the food processor when you start pulsing.

Serving Tip: I like to pair this with the Smothered Pork Chops (page 90). I even top the mash with some of the gravy made for the pork chops.

Macronutrients: 83% Fat, 6% Protein, 11% Carbs

Per serving: Calories: 227; Total Fat: 22g; Protein: 4g; Total Carbohydrates: 7g; Fiber: 2g; Erythritol: 0g; Net Carbs: 5g

Faux-tato Salad

NUT FREE

Serves 4
Prep Time: 20 minutes,
plus 1 hour to chill
Cook Time: 10 minutes

½ **head cauliflower, cut
into florets**

⅓ **cup mayonnaise**

2 **tablespoons
stone-ground mustard**

1 **tablespoon red
wine vinegar**

¼ **teaspoon pink Himalayan
sea salt**

¼ **teaspoon freshly ground
black pepper**

4 **ounces (5 to 6 strips)
bacon, cooked until crisp
and chopped**

1 **large egg, hard-boiled,
peeled, and chopped**

¼ **medium red onion,
thinly sliced**

2 **tablespoons grated
cheddar cheese**

2 **scallions, white and
green parts, chopped**

This ketogenic take on potato salad offers all the traditional flavors but without the carbs. It starts with fresh cauliflower cooked until fork-tender, which is then mixed with bacon, onion, egg, and cheese and blended with a creamy dressing.

1. Set a steamer basket in a small pot and add a couple inches of water. Place the cauliflower in the steamer, cover the pot, and steam for 7 to 10 minutes, until tender but not mushy. Let cool.

2. In a small bowl, combine the mayonnaise, mustard, vinegar, salt, and pepper.

3. In a large bowl, combine the cauliflower, bacon, chopped egg, red onion, cheese, and scallions.

4. Pour the dressing over the salad, then give it one final mix before serving. If desired, place the bowl in the refrigerator to chill the salad for about 1 hour before serving.

Cooking Tip: Fresh cauliflower works best for this, but you could use frozen. Simply cook it according to the package directions, then drain well.

Serving Tip: This recipe pairs great with the Jamaican Jerk Chicken (page 69). Since the chicken packs a little bit of spice, this salad offers a cool contrast.

Macronutrients: 86% Fat, 10% Protein, 4% Carbs

Per serving: Calories: 287; Total Fat: 27g; Protein: 7g; Total Carbohydrates: 3g; Fiber: 1g; Erythritol: 0g; Net Carbs: 2g

Garlic and Mozzarella Roasted Asparagus

EGG FREE, NUT FREE, UNDER 30 MINUTES, VEGETARIAN

Serves 2
Prep Time: 5 minutes
Cook Time: 15 minutes

2 tablespoons extra-virgin
   olive oil
1 garlic clove, minced
½ teaspoon pink Himalayan
   sea salt
¼ teaspoon freshly ground
   black pepper
8 ounces asparagus spears,
   bottoms trimmed
½ cup shredded
   low-moisture mozzarella

Asparagus is an underrated vegetable that offers so many preparation possibilities. Here you simply roast the asparagus in a bit of olive oil and top it with melty mozzarella cheese. The result is asparagus that maintains its natural snap with a subtle garlic flavor.

1. Preheat the oven to 425°F. Line a baking sheet with aluminum foil.

2. In a large bowl, combine the olive oil, garlic, salt, and pepper.

3. Add the asparagus to the bowl, then toss to coat in the oil mixture.

4. Transfer the asparagus to the baking sheet. Drizzle any remaining oil over the asparagus. Bake for 5 minutes.

5. Sprinkle the mozzarella evenly across the tips of the asparagus. Continue baking for an additional 5 to 7 minutes, until the cheese is slightly browned.

6. Transfer to serving plates and enjoy.

Serving Tip: This asparagus goes well with the Salmon Oscar (page 107). I place a layer of this asparagus on the serving plate, then put the salmon on top.

Macronutrients: 74% Fat, 15% Protein, 11% Carbs

Per serving: Calories: 229; Total Fat: 19g; Protein: 10g; Total Carbohydrates: 7g; Fiber: 2g; Erythritol: 0g; Net Carbs: 5g

Creamed Spinach

EGG FREE, NUT FREE, ONE PAN, UNDER 30 MINUTES, VEGETARIAN

Serves 2
Prep Time: 5 minutes
Cook Time: 10 minutes

2 tablespoons butter

6 ounces fresh
spinach, trimmed

¼ medium onion, chopped

2 garlic cloves, minced

½ cup heavy
(whipping) cream

¼ cup shredded
low-moisture
mozzarella cheese

¼ cup grated
Parmesan cheese

½ teaspoon pink Himalayan
sea salt

¼ teaspoon ground
white pepper

Creamed spinach is one of my favorite side dishes. Here it is lightly wilted and blended with a slightly peppery cream sauce. While the initial flavor comes from the Parmesan in the sauce, the spinach taste shines when paired with the unique flavor of white pepper.

1. In a large sauté pan or skillet, melt the butter over medium heat.

2. Add the spinach and onion. Stir and cook until the spinach is almost all wilted and the onion is translucent. Add the garlic and cook for an additional minute.

3. Using a slotted spoon, transfer the spinach to a bowl; leave the cooking juices in the skillet.

4. Add the cream, mozzarella, Parmesan, salt, and white pepper to the skillet. Stir with a wooden spoon until well blended.

5. Return the spinach to the skillet and stir to combine. Stirring gently, cook until the sauce thickens to your liking, then serve.

Serving Tip: This side dish pairs well with the Garlic Steak Bites (page 82). The dishes complement each other nicely—in fact, I've been known to dip a steak bite into the creamed spinach from time to time.

Macronutrients: 82% Fat, 10% Protein, 8% Carbs

Per serving: Calories: 433; Total Fat: 40g; Protein: 11g; Total Carbohydrates: 10g; Fiber: 2g; Erythritol: 0g; Net Carbs: 8g

Cauliflower French Fries

VEGETARIAN

Serves 2
Prep Time: 5 minutes,
plus 2 hours to freeze
Cook Time: 15 minutes

1 (8-ounce) package fresh
or frozen cauliflower rice

2 ounces full-fat
cream cheese

½ cup lupin flour (see Tip)

¼ cup grated
Parmesan cheese

1 large egg

1 tablespoon extra-virgin
olive oil

½ teaspoon pink Himalayan
sea salt

¼ teaspoon freshly ground
black pepper

If you thought you'd never have French fries again now that you're on the keto diet, think again! For this ketogenic take on the French fry, we turn to our old friend, cauliflower. A cauliflower mash plus a few other ingredients creates the perfect keto French fry. You get the fantastic crunch on the outside and the soft and almost creamy consistency inside. These fries also hold up well to a good dipping sauce.

1. Cook the cauliflower rice according to the package directions, then drain well. Unwrap the cream cheese, place in a microwave-safe bowl, and microwave on high power for 15 to 20 seconds.

2. In a food processor, combine the cauliflower and the melted cream cheese, the lupin flour, Parmesan, egg, olive oil, salt, and pepper. Blend on high speed until a paste forms. Be sure to scrape down the sides of the bowl from time to time.

3. Transfer the mixture to a resealable 1-gallon plastic bag, then cut a small bit off the corner of the bag. You want the opening to be between ¼ and ½ inch in diameter when spread open.

4. Line a large baking sheet with parchment paper.

5. Begin piping strips of the cauliflower mixture onto the baking sheet as close together as possible without their touching. (This may take some practice and the first ones might be rough; don't worry, they'll still taste great.)

CONTINUES ▶

6. Place the baking sheet in the freezer for at least 2 hours. (After 2 hours, the fries can be transferred to a freezer bag and stored for later use.)

7. Preheat the oven to 400°F.

8. Place a baking rack on a baking sheet. Place the fries in a single layer on the rack.

9. Bake the fries for 12 to 15 minutes, depending on size. You'll know they're done when the tips turn a darker shade of brown and the entire fry is golden brown. You can also touch one to check for crispiness. The fries should release easily from the baking rack. If the fry feels soft and is stuck to the rack, bake a bit longer and try again.

Ingredient Tip: Lupin flour is made from the sweet lupin bean and is very low in net carbs, due to its high fiber content. Lupin flour gives a smooth texture to the finished product, but if you're unable to find it, substitute almond flour.

Serving Tip: This side pairs well with the Crispy Chicken Tenders (page 71).

Macronutrients: 70% Fat, 23% Protein, 7% Carbs

Per serving: Calories: 400; Total Fat: 30g; Protein: 22g; Total Carbohydrates: 20g; Fiber: 14g; Net Carbs: 6g

Broccoli Fritters

NUT FREE, UNDER 30 MINUTES, VEGETARIAN

Serves 2
Prep Time: 10 minutes
Cook Time: 15 minutes

1 cup chopped
   broccoli florets
¼ cup almond flour
1 large egg
1 tablespoon grated
   Parmesan cheese
1 garlic clove, minced
½ teaspoon pink Himalayan
   sea salt
1 tablespoon extra-virgin
   olive oil
Sour cream (optional)

These broccoli fritters make a great side for any meal, but they can double as a keto vegetarian meal. The broccoli flavor is the focus here, but you'll pick up a hint of garlic and Parmesan cheese. While the taste might be unique, the texture is similar to potato pancakes; in fact, I eat them the same way, with a dollop of sour cream and some fresh chives on top.

1. Fill a large pot with about 1 inch of water, then fit with a steamer basket. Heat over medium-high heat until the water begins to simmer. Add the broccoli to the basket, cover the pot, and steam for 5 to 7 minutes, until the florets are tender.

2. In a food processor, combine the almond flour, egg, Parmesan, garlic, and salt. Pulse until the mixture is well blended.

3. Add the broccoli and pulse to incorporate. You want to have plenty of chunks.

4. In a griddle pan, heat the olive oil over medium-high heat. Spoon the broccoli onto the griddle in 2 portions, much like pancakes.

5. Cook for 4 to 5 minutes on each side, then serve with a side of sour cream, if desired.

Serving Tip: If you're eating this as a side dish, consider pairing it with the Parmesan-Crusted Salmon (page 98).

Macronutrients: 72% Fat, 15% Protein, 13% Carbs

Per serving: Calories: 193; Total Fat: 16g; Protein: 8g; Total Carbohydrates: 7g; Fiber: 3g; Erythritol: 0g; Net Carbs: 4g

Tomato and Artichoke Mushroom Pizzas

EGG FREE, NUT FREE, VEGETARIAN

Serves 2
Prep Time: 10 minutes
Cook Time: 20 minutes

2 large portobello
mushroom caps

¼ cup tomato sauce

½ teaspoon Italian
seasoning

¼ teaspoon pink Himalayan
sea salt

½ cup shredded
low-moisture
mozzarella cheese

2 tablespoons chopped
canned artichoke hearts

¼ cup halved cherry
tomatoes

Whether or not you're looking for a vegetarian option, pizzas made with the cap of a large portobello mushroom are a fantastic keto choice. The artichoke hearts and tomatoes are embedded in a gooey layer of melted cheese, giving every bite the perfect balance of earthiness, cheese flavor, and acidity.

1. Preheat the oven to 350°F. Line a baking sheet with aluminum foil.

2. Place the mushroom caps upside down on the baking sheet.

3. In a small bowl, combine the tomato sauce, Italian seasoning, and salt. Split the sauce between the 2 mushroom caps.

4. Add 2 tablespoons of the mozzarella to each cap.

5. Top the cheese with artichoke hearts and cherry tomatoes. Sprinkle the remaining ¼ cup mozzarella over the tops.

6. Bake for 20 minutes, until the cheese is melted, then serve.

Variation Tip: If you want to add some meat to this pizza, I recommend cooked ground chicken. It's a great way to put a new twist on this pizza.

Macronutrients: 45% Fat, 29% Protein, 26% Carbs

Per serving: Calories: 121; Total Fat: 6g; Protein: 10g; Total Carbohydrates: 9g; Fiber: 3g; Erythritol: 0g; Net Carbs: 6g

Sun-Dried Tomato and Pesto Zoodles

EGG FREE, ONE PAN, UNDER 30 MINUTES, VEGETARIAN

Serves 2
Prep Time: 5 minutes
Cook Time: 10 minutes

2 tablespoons extra-virgin
olive oil
2 medium zucchini,
spiralized
2 tablespoons basil pesto
2 tablespoons chopped
sun-dried tomatoes
2 tablespoons grated
Parmesan cheese

Pesto is an amazing source of flavor and healthy fats. Here, the pesto shines alongside the mild flavor of the zucchini noodles. Sun-dried tomatoes are added to give a nice burst of sweetness. And since no pesto dish would be complete without Parmesan cheese, there's plenty to sprinkle on top.

1. In a medium sauté pan or skillet, heat the olive oil over medium heat. Add the zucchini noodles and cook for about 5 minutes, until slightly soft; you want to retain some firmness.

2. Stir in the pesto, tomatoes, and Parmesan.

3. Gently stir to coat the zucchini with the pesto, then serve immediately.

Serving Tip: This recipe pairs great with any of the poultry dishes in this book. In fact, the combination of pesto and poultry is phenomenal, amplifying both dishes.

Macronutrients: 80% Fat, 7% Protein, 13% Carbs

Per serving: Calories: 268; Total Fat: 24g; Protein: 6g; Total Carbohydrates: 9g; Fiber: 3g; Erythritol: 0g; Net Carbs: 6g

Cauliflower "Mac" and Cheese

EGG FREE, NUT FREE, UNDER 30 MINUTES, VEGETARIAN

Serves 4
Prep Time: 5 minutes
Cook Time: 20 minutes

1 head of cauliflower
2 tablespoons butter
1 cup heavy
   (whipping) cream
2 ounces full-fat
   cream cheese
2 tablespoons sour cream
½ teaspoon pink Himalayan
   sea salt
½ teaspoon freshly ground
   black pepper
¼ teaspoon garlic powder
¼ teaspoon onion powder
¼ teaspoon red
   pepper flakes
1 cup shredded
   cheddar cheese

Who doesn't love a good mac and cheese? This recipe brings all the comfort of the childhood favorite to the ketogenic diet. The sauce is thick and creamy, and the cauliflower serves as a great pasta substitute.

1. Preheat the oven to 350°F.

2. Remove the leaves and core from the cauliflower, and cut the florets into bite-size pieces.

3. Fill a large pot with about 1 inch of water, then fit with a steamer basket. Heat over medium-high heat until the water begins to simmer. Add the cauliflower to the basket, cover the pot and steam for 7 to 9 minutes, until the florets are tender.

4. In a medium saucepan, melt the butter over medium heat. Add the cream, cream cheese, sour cream, salt, pepper, garlic powder, onion powder, and red pepper flakes. Stir with a wooden spoon until everything is well blended.

5. Add the cheddar in 2 portions, stirring well to allow the cheese to melt before adding more.

6. Place the cauliflower in an 8-inch square baking dish.

7. Pour the cheese sauce over the top, then bake for 10 minutes, until the sauce is bubbling.

Serving Tip: This recipe pairs great with the Breaded Pork Chops (page 95). Served alongside the crisped pork chops, this "mac" and cheese offers a fantastic balance of crispy and creamy.

Macronutrients: 85% Fat, 9% Protein, 6% Carbs

Per serving: Calories: 460; Total Fat: 42g; Protein: 10g; Total Carbohydrates: 10g; Fiber: 3g; Erythritol: 0g; Net Carbs: 6g

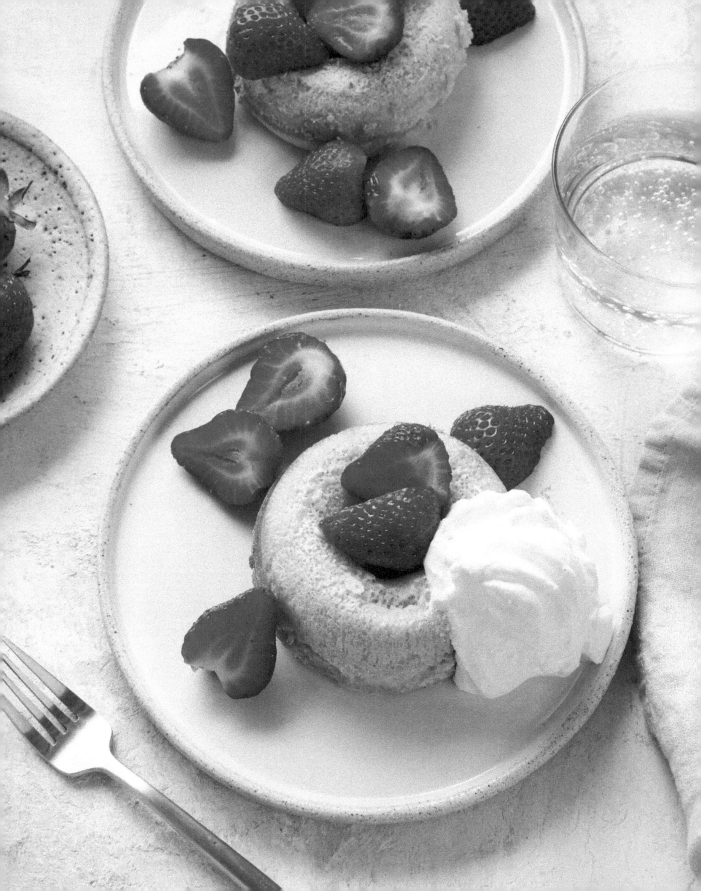

CHAPTER NINE

Desserts and Drinks

Chocolate Almond Smoothie

EGG FREE, UNDER 30 MINUTES, VEGETARIAN

Serves 2
Prep Time: 5 minutes

2 cups ice cubes

1 cup heavy
   (whipping) cream

1 cup water

¼ cup canned
   coconut cream

3 tablespoons
   almond butter

2 tablespoons
   cocoa powder

½ teaspoon liquid stevia

This can best be described as a liquid almond buttercup. The initial chocolatey flavor of every sip quickly turns into a subtle almond butter finish. The cold and creamy texture makes this sweet treat perfect for a hot summer's evening.

In a high-speed blender, combine the ice cubes, cream, water, coconut cream, almond butter, cocoa powder, and stevia. Blend on high speed until the mixture is smooth, then serve immediately.

Variation Tip: If you choose to drink alcohol, this is a great base for a cocktail. Reduce the water to ½ cup, then add ½ cup vodka or rum.

Macronutrients: 88% Fat, 5% Protein, 7% Carbs

Per serving: Calories: 669; Total Fat: 68g; Protein: 10g; Total Carbohydrates: 13g; Fiber: 5g; Erythritol: 1g; Net Carbs: 8g

Chocolate Chip Cookies

UNDER 30 MINUTES, VEGETARIAN

Makes 4 cookies
Prep Time: 5 minutes
Cook Time: 15 minutes

¼ cup (½ stick) butter, at
   room temperature
¼ cup granulated erythritol
¼ cup brown erythritol
1 large egg
½ teaspoon vanilla extract
1 cup almond flour
1 teaspoon xanthan gum
1 teaspoon baking powder
¼ teaspoon pink Himalayan
   sea salt
½ cup sugar-free
   chocolate chips

This recipe for classic chocolate chip cookies will remind you of the ones your mom used to make—except here you get four large, golden brown cookies that are moist, sweet, and of course, very low in carbs.

1. Preheat the oven to 375°F. Line a baking sheet with parchment paper.

2. In a large bowl, combine the butter, both erythritols, egg, and vanilla. Using a whisk or electric mixer on medium-high speed, cream the mixture until smooth.

3. In a medium bowl, combine the almond flour, xanthan gum, baking powder, and salt. Mix well, then add the dry ingredients to the wet ingredients and mix until well combined.

4. Fold in the chocolate chips.

5. Divide the dough into 4 equal portions and roll them into balls.

6. Flatten the balls to between ¼- and ½-inch thickness on the baking sheet. The dough will not spread when baking, so be sure they are flat enough.

7. Bake for 13 to 15 minutes, until golden brown.

8. Allow the cookies to cool on the baking sheet for 15 to 20 minutes, then cool further on a rack.

Macronutrients: 94% Fat, 2% Protein, 4% Carbs

Per cookie: Calories: 316; Total Fat: 33g; Protein: 7g; Total Carbohydrates: 5g; Fiber: 4g; Erythritol: 36g; Net Carbs: 1g

Keto Fudge

EGG FREE, NUT FREE, VEGETARIAN

Makes 4 pieces
Prep Time: 5 minutes,
plus 2 hours to chill
Cook Time: 20 minutes

1 cup heavy
  (whipping) cream
¾ teaspoon liquid stevia
Pinch of pink Himalayan
  sea salt
1 cup sugar-free
  semi-sweet baking chips
¼ cup chopped walnuts
  (optional)

This keto fudge is a longstanding crowd favorite. The texture and taste are practically indistinguishable from the real deal. It's firm and won't stick to your fingers, but is still smooth and creamy. Though the walnuts are optional, they add a nutty crunch.

1. In a medium saucepan, combine the cream, stevia, and salt. Whisk slowly over medium-low heat until the mixture comes to a boil. The initial boil can produce a lot of bubbles, so keep stirring to prevent it from overflowing.

2. Continue stirring until the mixture is reduced by half, about 15 minutes. Transfer to a large bowl and let cool.

3. Place the chocolate chips in a medium microwave-safe bowl. Microwave on high power for 30 seconds, then stir. Continue to microwave in 30-second intervals, stirring between each interval, until the chips are liquid. Be careful not to overdo it, or the chocolate may seize.

4. Slowly pour the melted chocolate into the cream mixture, whisking. Add the chopped walnuts, if using, and stir just enough to distribute the walnuts.

5. Line a small 8-inch loaf pan with parchment paper, and pour the fudge into the pan. Use a rubber scraper to spread the fudge evenly.

6. Refrigerate for 1 to 2 hours, until the fudge is firm.

7. For best results, remove the fudge from the refrigerator and let it rest on the counter for an additional 1 to 2 hours.

8. Cut into 4 squares and serve.

> **Cooking Tip:** If you prefer not to use a microwave to melt the chocolate chips, a double boiler is a great alternative, as is a water bath. You can create the water bath by placing about 1 inch of water in a medium saucepan, then positioning a large bowl with the chocolate atop the water but not touching. When the water is simmering, the steam will melt the chocolate in the bowl. Just remember to keep stirring.

> **Storage Tip:** Leftover fudge can be stored in an airtight container on the counter for up to 3 days or in the refrigerator for up to 1 week.

Macronutrients: 94% Fat, 4% Protein, 2% Carbs

Per piece: Calories: 308; Total Fat: 32g; Protein: 3g; Total Carbohydrates: 2g; Fiber: 0g; Erythritol: 12g; Net Carbs: 2g

Cheesecake

VEGETARIAN

Serves 4
Prep Time: 10 minutes,
plus 1 hour to chill
Cook Time: 40 minutes

Cheesecake has always been one of my favorite desserts, so it was the first keto sweet I made. This version has a sweet and creamy filling and crust that really set it apart.

For the crust

⅔ cup almond flour

2 teaspoons granulated erythritol

¼ teaspoon psyllium husk powder

⅛ teaspoon ground cinnamon

2 tablespoons butter, melted

1½ teaspoons heavy (whipping) cream

For the filling

8 ounces full-fat cream cheese, at room temperature

1 large egg

2 tablespoons granulated erythritol

2 tablespoons sour cream

¼ teaspoon freshly squeezed lemon juice

½ teaspoon liquid stevia

Pinch of pink Himalayan sea salt

1. Preheat the oven to 325°F.

2. **To make the crust:** In a small bowl, combine the almond flour, erythritol, psyllium husk powder, and cinnamon.

3. Add the butter and cream and combine with a fork.

4. Transfer the mixture to a 7-inch springform pan.

5. Using a fork or your hands, pack the mixture against the bottom of the pan to form a crust. Do not put crust up the sides.

6. **To make the filling:** In a large mixing bowl, using a whisk or hand mixer on medium-high speed, combine the cream cheese, egg, erythritol, sour cream, lemon juice, stevia, and salt.

7. Pour the filling directly over the crust.

8. Bake for 38 to 40 minutes, until the very edges have a hint of brown.

9. Remove cheesecake from the oven and let cool for 1 hour. Release the springform pan and transfer the cheesecake to the refrigerator to chill for at least 1 hour.

10. Cut the cheesecake into 4 pieces and serve.

Macronutrients: 84% Fat, 9% Protein, 7% Carbs

Per serving: Calories: 373; Total Fat: 36g; Protein: 9g; Total Carbohydrates: 6g; Fiber: 2g; Erythritol: 9g; Net Carbs: 4g

Birthday Mug Cakes

ONE PAN, UNDER 30 MINUTES, VEGETARIAN

Serves 2
Prep Time: 5 minutes
Cook Time: 2 minutes

For the frosting

2 ounces full-fat cream
cheese, at room
temperature

1 tablespoon butter, at
room temperature

2 teaspoons granulated
erythritol

¼ teaspoon vanilla extract

For the cake

⅓ cup almond flour

2 tablespoons granulated
erythritol

½ teaspoon baking powder

1 large egg

¼ teaspoon vanilla extract

Your birthday doesn't have to be a reason to blow your diet. With this keto birthday cake, you can have your cake and eat it, too. The cake resembles a small yellow cupcake, but is made quickly in the microwave. It is then topped with a cream cheese frosting. It might be tempting to eat the whole thing yourself, but I recommend sharing it with your diet partner.

1. **To make the frosting:** In a small bowl, combine the cream cheese, butter, erythritol, and vanilla. Whisk well, then place in the refrigerator to chill.

2. **To make the cake:** In a 12-ounce coffee mug, combine the almond flour, erythritol, and baking powder. Using a fork, break up any clumps and mix the ingredients well.

3. Add the egg and vanilla, then beat well. Make sure you scrape the bottom edges for any unmixed flour.

4. Microwave on high power for 70 seconds.

5. Let the cake cool for 5 to 10 minutes.

6. Flip the mug onto a plate, then tap a few times. (Alternately, you can skip this step and eat it directly from the mug.). Cut the cake in half crosswise, for 2 cupcakes.

7. Frost the cupcakes before serving.

Macronutrients: 81% Fat, 12% Protein, 7% Carbs

Per serving: Calories: 279; Total Fat: 26g; Protein: 8g; Total Carbohydrates: 5g; Fiber: 2g; Erythritol: 16g; Net Carbs: 3g

Chocolate Mousse

NUT FREE, VEGETARIAN

Serves 4
Prep Time: 10 minutes,
plus 2 hours to chill

1½ cups heavy (whipping)
cream, divided
1 cup sugar-free semisweet
baking chips
1 large egg yolk
1 teaspoon vanilla extract
¼ teaspoon liquid stevia

This recipe offers all the chocolatey flavors of a traditional mousse without the sugars. The dessert is sweet, with the slight bitterness of the chocolate shining through.

1. In a medium saucepan over medium-low heat, heat ½ cup of cream until it barely reaches a simmer. Add the chocolate chips and begin stirring. As soon as the chocolate is completely melted, remove the mixture from the heat.

2. In a small bowl, lightly beat the egg yolk, then add a few spoonfuls of the melted chocolate to warm the egg.

3. While whisking, stir the egg yolk into the chocolate in the saucepan. Let cool slightly.

4. In a medium bowl, mix the remaining 1 cup of cream, the vanilla, and stevia. Using an electric mixer on high speed or a whisk, beat for 5 to 7 minutes, until soft peaks form.

5. Pour the chocolate mixture over the whipped cream and gently fold in, using a rubber spatula and scraping down the sides of the bowl.

6. Pour the mousse into 4 serving bowls or ramekins. Refrigerate for 1 to 2 hours to set the mousse, then serve.

Ingredient Tip: Not all chocolate chips are keto friendly. I recommend Lily's, but any chocolate chips sweetened with stevia and/or erythritol will do.

Macronutrients: 85% Fat, 6% Protein, 9% Carbs

Per serving: Calories: 581; Total Fat: 55g; Protein: 8g; Total Carbohydrates: 14g; Fiber: 7g; Erythritol: 24g; Net Carbs: 7g

Cookies-and-Cream Fat Bomb

EGG FREE, NUT FREE, VEGETARIAN

Serves 2
Prep Time: 10 minutes,
plus 45 minutes to chill
Cook Time: 1 to 3 minutes

1¾ ounces cacao butter

4 teaspoons powdered
    erythritol

4 teaspoons heavy
    cream powder

Pinch of pink Himalayan
    sea salt

2 teaspoons cacao nibs

While most of my desserts fall into the category of a fat bomb, this one is special. The cookies and cream are a high-fat, very low-carb treat you can use to boost your fat intake on days when you've run out of other macros but still need some calories. The fat bomb itself will remind you of a cookies-and-cream candy bar, but it has a slightly more chocolatey note from the cacao nibs and cacao butter.

1. In a small microwave-safe bowl, heat the cacao butter on high power in 30-second increments until it is liquid. Make sure to stir between intervals of microwaving.

2. Add the powdered erythritol, heavy cream powder, and salt to the cacao butter. Whisk until the mixture is well combined.

3. Line 2 cups of a muffin pan with paper cupcake liners. Split the liquid between the cups.

4. Pour 1 teaspoon of cacao nibs into each cup, then place the muffin pan in the refrigerator to cool for about 1 hour. (The cups can be stored in the refrigerator until ready to enjoy.)

Cooking Tip: If you do not use a microwave, you can melt the cacao butter in a double boiler or water bath; for the latter, see the instructions on page 131.

Macronutrients: 89% Fat, 3% Protein, 8% Carbs

Per serving: Calories: 242; Total Fat: 24g; Protein: 1g; Total Carbohydrates: 5g; Fiber: 1g; Erythritol: 8g; Net Carbs: 4g

Mixed Berry Cobbler

EGG FREE, VEGETARIAN

Serves 4
Prep Time: 10 minutes
Cook Time: 35 minutes

For the filling

2 cups frozen mixed berries

1 tablespoon granulated
  erythritol

½ teaspoon water

¼ teaspoon freshly
  squeezed lemon juice

¼ teaspoon vanilla extract

For the crust

½ cup coconut flour

2 tablespoons granulated
  erythritol

½ teaspoon xanthan gum

½ teaspoon baking powder

6 tablespoons butter, cold

¼ cup heavy
  (whipping) cream

This mixed berry cobbler looks much harder to make than it actually is. The resulting dessert looks beautiful and is full of fresh flavor. The mixed berries are fine on their own, but here they are complemented with a hint of vanilla and lemon. The topping adds some buttery sweetness, so every bite is a perfect balance of sweet and tart.

1. Preheat the oven to 350°F.

2. **To make the filling:** In a 9-inch round pie dish, combine the berries, erythritol, water, lemon juice, and vanilla.

3. **To make the crust:** In a food processor, pulse to combine the coconut flour, erythritol, xanthan gum, and baking powder.

4. Add the butter and cream, and pulse until pea-sized pieces of dough form. Don't overprocess.

5. Form 5 equal balls of dough, then flatten them to between ¼- and ½-inch thickness.

6. Place the dough rounds on the top of the berries so that they are touching, but not overlapping.

1 teaspoon granulated
   erythritol

¼ teaspoon ground
   cinnamon

7. **To make the topping:** In a small bowl, combine the erythritol and cinnamon. Sprinkle the mixture over the dough.

8. Bake for 30 to 35 minutes, until the topping is beginning to brown, then let cool for 10 minutes before serving.

Storage Tip: Since this recipe makes 4 servings, you'll likely want to store leftovers in the refrigerator for up to 3 days. This dish is also great when served cold.

Macronutrients: 71% Fat, 5% Protein, 24% Carbs

Per serving: Calories: 317; Total Fat: 25g; Protein: 4g; Total Carbohydrates: 19g; Fiber: 7g; Erythritol: 10g; Net Carbs: 12g

Strawberry Shortcake

VEGETARIAN

Serves 3
Prep Time: 5 minutes,
plus 15 minutes to cool
Cook Time: 20 minutes

Coconut oil cooking spray
½ cup almond flour
¼ cup granulated erythritol
¼ teaspoon baking powder
3 large eggs
¼ teaspoon vanilla extract
¼ cup heavy
  (whipping) cream
⅛ teaspoon liquid stevia
Dash of vanilla extract
9 fresh strawberries, halved

My favorite strawberry shortcake is made with those small round sponge cakes sold in grocery stores. This keto version re-creates those sweet and fluffy cakes, then fills the centers with fresh strawberries and homemade whipped cream.

1. Preheat the oven to 350°F. Coat 3 molds of a donut pan with the cooking spray.

2. In a large bowl, combine the almond flour, erythritol, and baking powder. Whisk to break up any clumps.

3. In a small bowl, beat the eggs with the vanilla. Pour the wet ingredients into the dry ingredients and whisk to combine.

4. Fill the molds of the donut pan to the rim with the batter. You want to fill it all the way in order to get the bottom to close.

5. Bake for 15 to 17 minutes, until golden brown and a toothpick inserted into the center comes out clean.

6. Let the cakes cool for 15 minutes before attempting to remove them; otherwise, they may fall apart. Allowing them to completely cool is best.

7. In a medium bowl, combine the cream, stevia, and vanilla. Using a hand mixer on high speed or a whisk, beat vigorously for 5 to 7 minutes, until soft peaks form, or keep going to make a thicker whipped cream.

8. Place the cakes on serving plates. Fill each with 6 strawberry halves, then top with the whipped cream.

Variation Tip: For those people allergic to almonds, use ¼ cup coconut flour instead of the ½ cup almond flour. Coconut flour will absorb more liquid, so it may be necessary to thin the batter with a tablespoon or so of heavy (whipping) cream.

Macronutrients: 72% Fat, 17% Protein, 11% Carbs

Per serving: Calories: 245; Total Fat: 20g; Protein: 10g; Total Carbohydrates: 7g; Fiber: 3g; Erythritol: 16g; Net Carbs: 4g

Keto Mojito

DAIRY FREE, EGG FREE, NUT FREE, UNDER 30 MINUTES, VEGETARIAN

Makes 1 drink
Prep Time: 5 minutes

5 fresh mint leaves

1½ ounces (3 tablespoons) white rum

2 tablespoons freshly squeezed lime juice

1 tablespoon granulated erythritol

8 ounces soda water

Ice cubes

A mojito is a bright and refreshing cocktail that is both minty and citrusy. This keto version removes the carbs. The erythritol not only sweetens this drink—its mildly minty aftertaste also complements the flavors of this cocktail.

1. In a large, sturdy glass, muddle the mint leaves with either a muddler or the back of a spoon.

2. Add the rum, lime juice, and erythritol. Stir until the erythritol dissolves.

3. Top with the soda water and ice cubes, then enjoy.

Macronutrients: 2% Fat, 6% Protein, 92% Carbs

Per serving: Calories: 105; Total Fat: 0g; Protein: 0g; Total Carbohydrates: 2g; Fiber: 0g; Erythritol: 12g; Net Carbs: 2g

Frozen Strawberry Margarita

DAIRY FREE, EGG FREE, NUT FREE, UNDER 30 MINUTES, VEGETARIAN

Serves 3
Prep Time: 5 minutes

1 (10-ounce) package frozen strawberries

4½ ounces (9 tablespoons) tequila

5½ tablespoons freshly squeezed lime juice

3 tablespoons granulated erythritol

⅛ teaspoon orange extract

When it comes to frozen cocktails, the margarita is king. This ketogenic take on the strawberry margarita offers the refreshing flavors of the drink without breaking the keto diet. The flavors of strawberry and lime are the first on your tongue, but you'll get a subtle hint of orange on the finish. Just remember, alcohol contains calories, and calories still count.

In a large blender, combine the strawberries, tequila, lime juice, erythritol, and orange extract, and run on high speed until the mixture is smooth. Pour into 3 large glasses, then serve.

Cooking Tip: If you desire a thicker drink, add some ice to the blend.

Macronutrients: 3% Fat, 4% Protein, 93% Carbs

Per serving: Calories: 138; Total Fat: 0g; Protein: 1g; Total Carbohydrates: 11g; Fiber: 3g; Erythritol: 12g; Net Carbs: 8g

Whiskey Sour

DAIRY FREE, EGG FREE, NUT FREE, UNDER 30 MINUTES, VEGETARIAN

Makes 1 drink
Prep Time: 2 minutes

1½ ounces (3 table-
    spoons) whiskey
2 tablespoons freshly
    squeezed lemon juice
2 tablespoons water
¼ teaspoon liquid stevia
Ice cubes

I'd almost written off whiskey sours when I started the keto diet. But you'd be surprised how easy it is to replicate the sweet and sour flavor in this cocktail. The cocktail is sweet, sour, and mildly boozy, all at once. Choose a good whiskey to highlight the flavor, and you'll be on your way to one delicious drink.

In a small glass, combine the whiskey, lemon juice, water, and stevia and mix well. Top with the ice cubes and serve.

Macronutrients: 9% Fat, 5% Protein, 86% Carbs

Per serving: Calories: 104; Total Fat: 0g; Protein: 0g; Total Carbohydrates: 2g; Fiber: 0g; Erythritol: 2g; Net Carbs: 2g

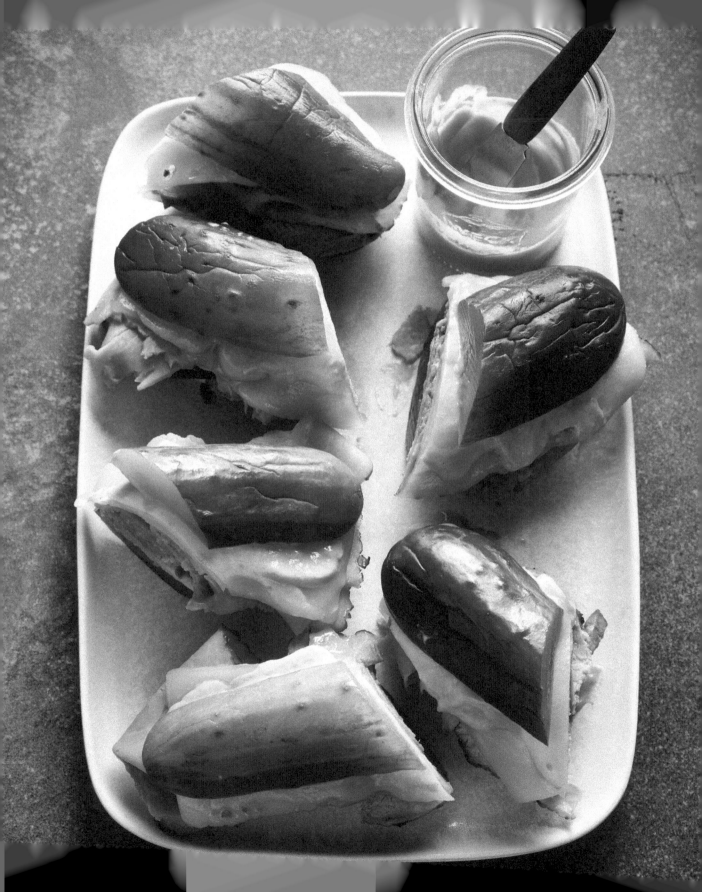

CHAPTER TEN

Snacks and Small Plates

Sausage-Stuffed Mushrooms

EGG FREE, NUT FREE

Serves 4
Prep Time: 15 minutes
Cook Time: 45 minutes

8 extra-large white
  button mushrooms,
  stems removed
3 tablespoons extra-virgin
  olive oil, divided
8 ounces ground spicy
  Italian sausage
¼ medium onion, chopped
1 garlic clove, minced
½ cup grated
  Parmesan cheese
2 ounces full-fat cream
  cheese, at room
  temperature
Pink Himalayan sea salt
Freshly ground
  black pepper

Whether for a snack or your contribution to the next pot-luck, these stuffed mushrooms will satisfy guests regardless of the diet they follow. The tender mushroom caps serve as the perfect delivery method for the spicy sausage stuffing. The heat is balanced by a blend of cheeses that coats the filling. When packed into the mushrooms along with garlic and onion, the stuffed mushrooms are a perfect bite of food.

1. Preheat the oven to 325°F.

2. In a large bowl, toss the mushrooms with 2 table-spoons of olive oil.

3. In a medium sauté pan or skillet, heat the remaining tablespoon of olive oil over medium-high heat. Add the sausage and cook for 4 to 5 minutes, until browned.

4. Add the onion and garlic and cook for an additional 5 minutes, until the onion is translucent.

5. Add the Parmesan cheese and cream cheese. Keep stirring until the cream cheese has coated the meat and the Parmesan is just starting to melt. Season with salt and pepper.

6. Distribute the meat mixture among the mushrooms, mounding the filling in the centers. Place them in an 8-inch or larger square baking dish.

7. Bake for 45 minutes, then cool briefly and serve.

Storage Tip: These stuffed mushrooms reheat surprisingly well. Store them in an airtight container in the refrigerator for up to 3 days, then reheat in the microwave when you're ready to eat them.

Macronutrients: 81% Fat, 14% Protein, 5% Carbs

Per serving: Calories: 401; Total Fat: 36g; Protein: 14g; Total Carbohydrates: 5g; Fiber: 1g; Erythritol: 0g; Net Carbs: 4g

Jalapeño Poppers

EGG FREE, NUT FREE, UNDER 30 MINUTES

Serves 3
Prep Time: 5 minutes
Cook Time: 25 minutes

3 ounces full-fat cream
    cheese, at room
    temperature
¼ cup shredded
    cheddar cheese
⅛ teaspoon pink Himalayan
    sea salt
⅛ teaspoon freshly ground
    black pepper
Pinch of cayenne pepper
3 jalapeño
    peppers, stemmed
3 thick-cut bacon slices,
    halved lengthwise

This ketogenic, bacon-wrapped jalapeño popper has been a go-to of mine for years. While most poppers are just filled with cream cheese, this version uses a blend of cream cheese, cheddar cheese, and spices to produce a much more complex taste.

1. In a small bowl, combine the cream cheese, cheddar cheese, salt, pepper, and cayenne.

2. Preheat the oven to 400°F. Line a baking sheet with aluminum foil.

3. Slice the jalapeños in half lengthwise. Using a spoon, remove the seeds and membranes.

4. Fill each jalapeño half with an equal portion of the cheese mixture, then wrap it in the bacon strips. Use a toothpick to secure the bacon, if necessary.

5. Place the poppers on the prepared baking sheet and bake for 20 to 25 minutes, until the bacon is crisp and the jalapeño is tender. Let cool briefly, then serve.

Variation Tip: If you want some extra spice, finely mince some of the jalapeño membranes and seeds, then add to the cheese filling. Be careful how much you add, as jalapeños can vary quite a bit in heat.

Macronutrients: 78% Fat, 17% Protein, 5% Carbs

Per serving: Calories: 193; Total Fat: 17g; Protein: 8g; Total Carbohydrates: 2g; Fiber: 0g; Erythritol: 0g; Net Carbs: 2g

Deviled Eggs

DAIRY FREE, NUT FREE, UNDER 30 MINUTES, VEGETARIAN

Serves 2
Prep Time: 5 minutes
Cook Time: 15 minutes

4 large eggs
2 tablespoons mayonnaise
½ teaspoon
  whole-grain mustard
½ teaspoon apple
  cider vinegar
½ teaspoon dill relish
Pinch of cayenne pepper
Pink Himalayan sea salt
Freshly ground
  black pepper
Paprika, for garnish

Deviled eggs are a great snack for the keto diet. The protein and fat ratios are fantastic, and the carbs are incredibly low. These deviled eggs have a mild pickle flavor blended with the traditional mayonnaise and mustard dressing. Since hard-boiled eggs are easy to keep on hand, this snack can quickly become a staple.

1. Bring a medium pot with 2 to 3 inches of water to a rolling boil. Place the eggs in the pot and boil for 15 minutes.

2. Using a spoon, transfer the eggs to a large bowl with ice water to cool.

3. In a small bowl, combine the mayonnaise, mustard, vinegar, and relish. Season with the cayenne, salt, and pepper.

4. Peel the eggs and slice them in half lengthwise. Remove the yolks and add them to the bowl with the other ingredients. Using a fork, mash the yolks into the mayonnaise mixture to create the filling.

5. Fill the cavity of each egg with some of the filling.

6. Lightly sprinkle the tops of the eggs with paprika before serving.

Cooking Tip: Adding about 1 tablespoon vinegar to the boiling water will help the shells release easier.

Macronutrients: 75% Fat, 23% Protein, 2% Carbs

Per serving: Calories: 238; Total Fat: 20g; Protein: 13g; Total Carbohydrates: 1g; Fiber: 0g; Erythritol: 0g; Net Carbs: 1g

Spinach–Artichoke–Jalapeño Dip

EGG FREE, NUT FREE, UNDER 30 MINUTES, VEGETARIAN

Serves 4
Prep Time: 5 minutes
Cook Time: 15 minutes

¼ cup cooked fresh spinach or thawed frozen

½ cup grated Parmesan cheese

3 ounces full-fat cream cheese

⅓ cup canned artichoke hearts

2 tablespoons sour cream

2 tablespoons mayonnaise

1 jalapeño pepper, seeded and finely chopped

1 garlic clove, minced

½ teaspoon pink Himalayan sea salt

½ teaspoon freshly ground black pepper

This warm and creamy dip is best served with pork rinds or cheese crisps. Combine this with a slight heat from the jalapeño, and you'll wish you had made more.

1. Preheat the oven to 350°F.

2. In a medium bowl, combine the spinach, Parmesan, cream cheese, artichoke hearts, sour cream, mayonnaise, jalapeño, garlic, salt, and pepper and mix to combine.

3. Transfer the mixture to a ramekin or other small baking dish. Bake for 15 minutes, then serve.

Variation Tip: If you don't like spice, leave out the jalapeño. Conversely, if you want more heat, mince some of the seeds and membranes and add to the dip.

Macronutrients: 78% Fat, 12% Protein, 10% Carbs

Per serving: Calories: 196; Total Fat: 17g; Protein: 6g; Total Carbohydrates: 5g; Fiber: 2g; Erythritol: 0g; Net Carbs: 3g

Italian Pinwheels

NUT FREE, UNDER 30 MINUTES

Serves 2
Prep Time: 5 minutes

2 tablespoons mayonnaise

1 tablespoon extra-virgin
olive oil

1 tablespoon red
wine vinegar

½ teaspoon Italian
seasoning

2 Keto Tortillas (page 174),
cooled

4 deli pepperoni slices

4 deli salami slices

4 thin slices
cheddar cheese

2 iceberg lettuce leaves

As far as hors d'oeuvres go, a pinwheel is the perfect way to impress your guests without much effort. This Italian pinwheel wraps your favorite Italian deli meats with lettuce, cheese, and a mayonnaise-based sauce. When it's cut into bite-size pieces, you've got the ultimate finger food.

1. In a small bowl, mix the mayonnaise, olive oil, vinegar, and Italian seasoning. Spread the tortillas with the sauce.

2. Layer on the pepperoni, salami, cheese, and lettuce.

3. Roll the tortillas into tight cylinders, then place seam-side down on a cutting board.

4. If the wraps have loose ends, secure them with toothpicks spaced roughly 1 inch apart.

5. Cut the wraps into 1-inch pieces, then serve.

Prep Tip: Cheese does not like to roll, especially if it is cut into thick slices, so be sure to use thinly sliced cheese.

Macronutrients: 78% Fat, 12% Protein, 10% Carbs

Per serving: Calories: 610; Total Fat: 53g; Protein: 19g; Total Carbohydrates: 14g; Fiber: 7g; Erythritol: 0g; Net Carbs: 7g

Jumbo Pickle Cuban Sandwich

NUT FREE, EGG FREE, UNDER 30 MINUTES

Serves 2
Prep Time: 5 minutes
Cook Time: 5 minutes

2 deli ham slices

2 deli pork tenderloin slices

4 Swiss cheese slices

2 jumbo dill pickles, halved
   lengthwise (see Tip)

1 tablespoon
   yellow mustard

A Cuban sandwich is the perfect combination of ham, Swiss cheese, pickles, and mustard, melted into a delicious sandwich. This ketogenic take on a classic Cuban uses a jumbo pickle to replace the bread, but otherwise keeps all the flavors of the original.

1. In a small sauté pan or skillet, heat the ham and tenderloin slices over medium heat until warm.

2. Using a spatula, roll the deli meats into loose rolls. Top with the Swiss cheese slices and allow the cheese to begin to melt.

3. Transfer the rolls to 2 pickle halves.

4. Top the cheese with some mustard, then close the sandwiches by topping them with the matching pickle halves.

5. Secure with toothpicks and slice in half crosswise, then serve.

Ingredient Tip: Find the absolute biggest pickles that you can. For me, this usually means getting them individually wrapped from the grocery store or a gas station.

Macronutrients: 59% Fat, 39% Protein, 2% Carbs

Per serving: Calories: 256; Total Fat: 16g; Protein: 23g; Total Carbohydrates: 5g; Fiber: 4g; Erythritol: 0g; Net Carbs: 1g

Buffalo Chicken Dip

EGG FREE, NUT FREE

Serves 4
Prep Time: 5 minutes
Cook Time: 25 minutes

1 pound boneless, skinless chicken thighs

8 ounces full-fat cream cheese, at room temperature

¼ cup Garlic Ranch Dressing (page 163) or store-bought ranch dressing

¼ cup hot sauce of choice

¼ cup blue cheese crumbles

Whether it's game day or movie night at home, this buffalo chicken dip is the perfect snack. The tender chicken is suspended in a creamy buffalo ranch dressing. When served with crisp celery sticks, the result is the perfect balance of flavors and textures.

1. In a medium saucepan, cover the chicken thighs with water and poach for about 20 minutes, until the chicken is cooked through. Drain. Using 2 forks, shred the chicken.

2. Add the cream cheese, dressing, hot sauce, and blue cheese to the saucepan. Add the chicken. Stir while cooking over medium heat for about 5 minutes, until the ingredients are smoothly combined.

3. Serve with celery stalks or other snack of choice.

Storage Tip: This dip can be stored in an airtight container in the refrigerator for up to 5 days. As a bonus, it is also really good served cold.

Macronutrients: 70% Fat, 27% Protein, 3% Carbs

Per serving: Calories: 426; Total Fat: 33g; Protein: 28g; Total Carbohydrates: 3g; Fiber: 0g; Erythritol: 0g; Net Carbs: 3g

Pepperoni Pizza Bites

UNDER 30 MINUTES

Serves 4
Prep Time: 10 minutes
Cook Time: 15 minutes

Olive oil or coconut oil, for
    greasing
1 cup shredded
    low-moisture mozzarella
    cheese, divided
1 ounce full-fat cream
    cheese, at room
    temperature
⅓ cup almond flour
1 large egg
4 teaspoons keto
    marinara sauce
8 pepperoni slices

If you're looking for a great snack or small lunch, these keto pizza bites are perfect. Think of them as the keto equivalent of a bagel pizza, delivering on both portability and flavor. The crust crisps nicely on the edges while still staying soft in the middle; the topping is a keto marinara sauce with pepperoni and cheese. Don't feel limited by that, though—this crust will support anything you put on top of it.

1. Preheat the oven to 400°F. Grease 4 cups of a muffin pan with a little olive oil.

2. In a medium microwave-safe bowl, combine ¾ cup of mozzarella with the cream cheese.

3. Microwave on high power in 30-second increments until the cheeses are melted. Stir between intervals.

4. Add the almond flour and egg to the bowl and quickly mix. If the dough does not combine into a smooth texture, microwave for 10 to 15 seconds to soften it again before mixing.

5. Divide the dough into 4 portions.

6. Place a portion of dough into each muffin cup, then use a spoon to level the top. Make a depression in the center using the back of a spoon.

7. Bake for 7 minutes. Top each portion with 1 teaspoon marinara sauce, 1 tablespoon of mozzarella, and 2 pepperoni slices.

8. Bake for an additional 7 to 10 minutes, until the cheese is melted and the edges of the dough are browned.

9. Let the pizza bites cool for about 10 minutes, then remove from the pan and serve.

> **Cooking Tip:** Alternatively, you can melt the cheeses in a saucepan. Just be careful to remove the cheese from the heat before adding the egg so the egg does not cook during the mixing process.

Macronutrients: 70% Fat, 22% Protein, 8% Carbs

Per serving: Calories: 204; Total Fat: 16g; Protein: 12g; Total Carbohydrates: 4g; Fiber: 1g; Erythritol: 0g; Net Carbs: 3g

Bacon-Wrapped Pickle Fries

DAIRY FREE, EGG FREE, NUT FREE, ONE PAN, UNDER 30 MINUTES

Serves 3
Prep Time: 5 minutes
Cook Time: 25 minutes

6 dill pickle spears
6 bacon strips
Ranch dressing of choice

This might just be the most unusual recipe in this book, but it's here for a good reason. These bacon-wrapped pickle fries bring together a blend of flavors and textures that just simply works. The bacon provides salty crunch wrapped around a juicy dill pickle spear. It may be easy to make, but the dish is far from boring.

1. Preheat the oven to 425°F.

2. Wrap each pickle spear tightly with a strip of bacon. Secure the loose end of the bacon with a toothpick and place the spears on a small baking sheet.

3. Bake for 25 minutes, until the bacon is crispy. Let cool briefly, then serve with ranch dressing.

Variation Tip: Coating the pickles with a keto barbecue sauce (see page 165) for the last 10 minutes of cooking offers a variation on this snack. The sauce glazes the bacon and provides a subtle sweetness.

Macronutrients: 67% Fat, 26% Protein, 7% Carbs

Per serving (2 tablespoons): Calories: 97; Total Fat: 7g; Protein: 6g; Total Carbohydrates: 2g; Fiber: 1g; Erythritol: 0g; Net Carbs: 1g

Keto Trail Mix

EGG FREE, UNDER 5 MINUTES, UNDER 30 MINUTES, VEGETARIAN

Serves 4
Prep Time: 5 minutes

¼ cup pumpkin seeds

¼ cup salted almonds

¼ cup salted
  macadamia nuts

¼ cup salted walnuts

1 cup crunchy cheese snack
  (see Tip)

¼ cup sugar-free
  chocolate chips

Eating keto on-the-go has never been simpler. Simply toss some shelf-stable ingredients into a bag, shake it up, and you're ready to go. A good trail mix needs salt, sweet, and crunchy components. This one checks all the boxes, with crunch up front, followed by a salty sweet mix of nuts and chocolate.

In a resealable 1-quart plastic bag, combine the pumpkin seeds, almonds, macadamia nuts, walnuts, cheese snack, and chocolate chips. Seal the bag and shake to mix.

Storage Tip: You can store the trail mix in an airtight bag in the pantry for as long as the soonest expiration date on any of the ingredients.

Ingredient Tip: Crunchy cheese is a keto-friendly snack made of dehydrated cheese. My favorite brands are Moon Cheese and Intakt.

Macronutrients: 82% Fat, 11% Protein, 7% Carbs

Per serving: Calories: 253; Total Fat: 23g; Protein: 7g; Total Carbohydrates: 5g; Fiber: 3g; Erythritol: 8g; Net Carbs: 2g

Granola Clusters

DAIRY FREE, UNDER 30 MINUTES, VEGETARIAN

Serves 2
Prep Time: 5 minutes
Cook Time: 15 minutes

¼ cup almonds

¼ cup pecans

¼ cup macadamia nuts

1 large egg white

2 tablespoons ground
flaxseed

1 tablespoon coconut
oil, melted

1 tablespoon
pumpkin seeds

1 tablespoon chia seeds

1 tablespoon unsweetened
coconut flakes

1 tablespoon granulated
erythritol

¼ teaspoon vanilla extract

⅛ teaspoon pink Himalayan
sea salt

Granola has a variety of uses and this recipe is no different. The chewy yet crunchy blend of nuts, seeds, and coconut produces an all-around great-tasting granola. This version highlights the nuts and seeds without overpowering it with sweetness. While this is a great snack to grab and go, it also makes an amazing keto cereal or yogurt topping.

1. Preheat the oven to 325°F. Line a baking sheet with parchment paper.

2. In a food processor, combine the almonds, pecans, macadamia nuts, egg white, flaxseed, coconut oil, pumpkin seeds, chia seeds, coconut flakes, erythritol, vanilla, and salt. Pulse until the largest chunks of nuts are about the size of a pea.

3. Spread the mixture evenly on the baking sheet. Bake for 15 to 18 minutes, until the granola is lightly browned.

4. Let cool for about 20 minutes, then break into clusters.

Variation Tip: Once the granola has cooled, you can melt about ¼ cup sugar-free chocolate chips and drizzle the chocolate across the top to create a chocolate granola cluster.

Macronutrients: 79% Fat, 9% Protein, 13% Carbs

Per serving: Calories: 482; Total Fat: 45g; Protein: 12g; Total Carbohydrates: 15g; Fiber: 10g; Erythritol: 6g; Net Carbs: 5g

Cheese Crisps

DAIRY FREE, EGG FREE, NUT FREE, ONE PAN, VEGETARIAN

Serves 2
Prep Time: 2 minutes
Cook Time: 35 minutes

6 thin square slices
  of packaged
  cheddar cheese
Pinch of pink Himalayan
  sea salt

Here is a "keto hack" for you that will prove endlessly useful. When baked slowly at lower temperatures, cheese becomes crispy with a more concentrated flavor. Use this to your advantage, and create some amazing cheese crisps, or crackers. While this works with pretty much any cheese, the cheddar flavor concentrates nicely and the color is fantastic. Add a sprinkle of salt or your favorite spice blend before baking to create your own cheese cracker flavors.

1. Preheat the oven to 250°F. Line a baking sheet with parchment paper.

2. Cut each cheese slice into quarters.

3. Place the squares on the prepared baking sheet.

4. Sprinkle a little salt on each square.

5. Bake for 30 to 35 minutes, until the cheese starts to turn slightly brown.

6. Let cool for 10 minutes, then serve.

Ingredient Tip: Buying packaged thinly sliced cheese from the store is the way to go. It is very hard to get the slices thin enough when slicing by hand. If your slices are thicker, you can get a decent result, but the bake time will be longer.

Macronutrients: 74% Fat, 24% Protein, 2% Carbs

Per serving: Calories: 230; Total Fat: 19g; Protein: 14g; Total Carbohydrates: 1g; Fiber: 0g; Erythritol: 0g; Net Carbs: 1g

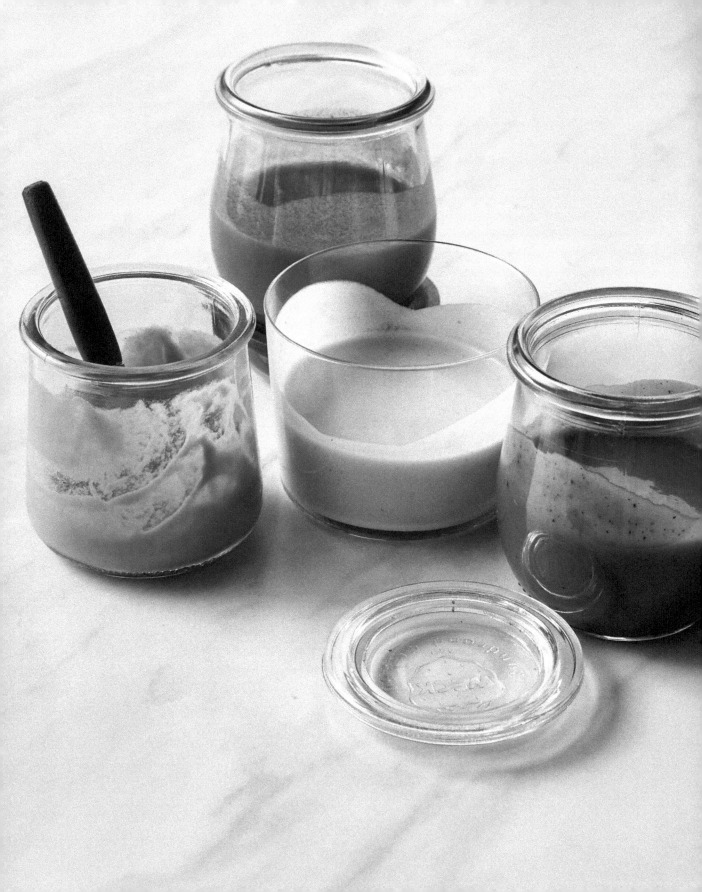

Sauces and Staples

Burger Sauce

DAIRY FREE, NUT FREE, ONE BOWL, UNDER 30 MINUTES, VEGETARIAN

Makes about ½ cup

Prep Time: 2 minutes

¼ cup mayonnaise

2 tablespoons
  sugar-free ketchup

2 tablespoons
  yellow mustard

1 tablespoon dill relish

If you're wondering what exactly a burger sauce is, you're probably not alone. This sauce combines all the ingredients that would be standard on a burger. But it doesn't stop there—the sauce can double as a salad dressing, a dipping sauce for fries and chicken tenders, or a steak sauce. While it may sound simple, having the ingredients already mixed produces a different flavor than adding them separately to your burger.

In a small bowl, combine the mayonnaise, ketchup, mustard, and relish; mix until well blended.

Storage Tip: Store this sauce in an airtight container in the refrigerator for up to 1 week.

Macronutrients: 94% Fat, 2% Protein, 4% Carbs

Per serving (2 tablespoons): Calories: 101; Total Fat: 11g; Protein: 1g; Total Carbohydrates: 1g; Fiber: 1g; Erythritol: 0g; Net Carbs: 0g

Garlic Ranch Dressing

NUT FREE, ONE BOWL, UNDER 30 MINUTES, VEGETARIAN

Makes ¾ cup
Prep Time: 5 minutes

¼ cup mayonnaise

¼ cup sour cream

2 tablespoons heavy (whipping) cream

2 tablespoons water

1 teaspoon freshly squeezed lemon juice

¾ teaspoon garlic powder

¼ teaspoon dried dill

¼ teaspoon dried parsley

¼ teaspoon dried chives

⅛ teaspoon onion powder

⅛ teaspoon pink Himalayan sea salt

⅛ teaspoon freshly ground black pepper

Most ranch dressings can be used on a ketogenic diet to some degree. Still, nothing beats the flavor of homemade ranch. Not only do you know exactly what's in it, but you can also adjust the ingredients to fit your taste! This keto ranch has a garlicky flavor, which makes it a great dipping sauce for everything from celery to keto pizza.

In a small bowl, whisk together the mayonnaise, sour cream, cream, water, lemon juice, garlic powder, dill, parsley, chives, onion powder, salt, and pepper. If possible, allow to sit for 30 minutes so the flavors can marry before serving.

Variation Tip: If you're looking for more of a traditional ranch dressing, reduce the garlic powder to ¼ teaspoon.

Storage Tip: Store this sauce in an airtight container in the refrigerator for up to 1 week.

Macronutrients: 95% Fat, 2% Protein, 3% Carbs

Per serving (2 tablespoons): Calories: 100; Total Fat: 11g; Protein: 0g; Total Carbohydrates: 1g; Fiber: 0g; Erythritol: 0g; Net Carbs: 1g

Cheese Sauce

EGG FREE, NUT FREE, ONE PAN, UNDER 30 MINUTES, VEGETARIAN

Makes about ½ cup
Prep Time: 5 minutes
Cook Time: 5 minutes

2 tablespoons sour cream

2 tablespoons heavy
(whipping) cream

¼ teaspoon pink Himalayan
sea salt

⅛ teaspoon freshly ground
black pepper

Pinch of garlic powder

Pinch of cayenne pepper

¼ cup grated
cheddar cheese

A good cheese sauce is a must for the keto diet. I use this sauce as a topping for vegetables and a dipping sauce for pork rinds. In fact, it tastes great on just about everything. Its flavor can best be described as a mild nacho cheese, a creamy sauce complemented by the sharpness of cheddar, garlic, and a touch of heat.

1. In a medium saucepan, heat the sour cream, cream, salt, pepper, garlic powder, and cayenne over medium heat.

2. Continue to stir until the sauce just begins to simmer.

3. Reduce the heat and slowly stir in the cheddar cheese.

4. When the cheese is blended into the sauce, serve immediately.

Macronutrients: 85% Fat, 12% Protein, 3% Carbs

Per serving (2 tablespoons): Calories: 66; Total Fat: 6g; Protein: 2g; Total Carbohydrates: 0g; Fiber: 0g; Erythritol: 0g; Net Carbs: 0g

Barbecue Sauce

DAIRY FREE, EGG FREE, NUT FREE, UNDER 30 MINUTES, VEGETARIAN

Makes about 1 cup
Prep Time: 5 minutes
Cook Time: 10 minutes

¾ cup sugar-free ketchup

3 tablespoons
allulose, divided

1 tablespoon apple
cider vinegar

1 teaspoon paprika

1 teaspoon onion powder

1 teaspoon freshly ground
black pepper

1 teaspoon spicy
whole-grain mustard

½ teaspoon
coconut aminos

¼ teaspoon liquid smoke

If you're missing that sweet, tangy flavor of barbecue sauce on your keto diet, you'll find this ketogenic version packs all the flavor of the traditional condiment, minus the carbs. While the sauce is sweet and tangy with a hint of pepper, no barbecue sauce would be complete without the mildly smoky undertone.

1. In a bowl, combine the ketchup, 2 tablespoons of allulose, the vinegar, paprika, onion powder, pepper, mustard, coconut aminos, and liquid smoke. Mix well, then transfer to a small saucepan.

2. Cook over medium-high heat for 3 to 5 minutes. The sauce should darken slightly.

3. Add the remaining tablespoon of allulose, then cook for an additional 1 to 2 minutes.

4. Let cool, then use as desired.

Storage Tip: Any unused sauce can be stored in an airtight container in the refrigerator for up to 1 week.

Macronutrients: 1% Fat, 2% Protein, 97% Carbs

Per serving (2 tablespoons): Calories: 10; Total Fat: 0g; Protein: 0g; Total Carbohydrates: 2g; Fiber: 1g; Erythritol: 0g; Allulose: 6g; Net Carbs: 1g

Marinara Sauce

EGG FREE, NUT FREE, ONE PAN, UNDER 30 MINUTES, VEGETARIAN

Makes about 2 cups
Prep Time: 5 minutes
Cook Time: 10 minutes

1 (15-ounce) can tomato sauce or puree
1 tablespoon grated Parmesan cheese
1 tablespoon extra-virgin olive oil
1 teaspoon minced garlic
1 teaspoon Italian seasoning
½ teaspoon pink Himalayan sea salt
¼ teaspoon red pepper flakes
⅛ teaspoon liquid stevia

Most store-bought jars of marinara are loaded with sugar. This ketogenic version is slightly sweet, mildly acidic, and full of your favorite Italian spices. Garlic and a hint of red pepper complete the sauce, with a balance of flavors. Whether you're putting it on zoodles or topping a pizza, this sauce can do it all.

1. In a small saucepan over low heat, combine the tomato sauce, Parmesan, olive oil, garlic, Italian seasoning, salt, red pepper flakes, and stevia over medium heat. Heat the mixture until it reaches a mild simmer.

2. Let the sauce simmer for about 10 minutes, stirring occasionally, until the flavors meld, then use as desired.

Storage Tip: Any leftover sauce can be stored in an airtight container in the refrigerator for up to 1 week.

Macronutrients: 46% Fat, 8% Protein, 46% Carbs

Per serving (½ cup): Calories: 77; Total Fat: 4g; Protein: 2g; Total Carbohydrates: 10g; Fiber: 2g; Erythritol: 0g; Net Carbs: 8g

"Honey" Mustard

DAIRY FREE, EGG FREE, NUT FREE, ONE BOWL, UNDER 30 MINUTES, VEGETARIAN

Makes ½ cup
Prep Time: 5 minutes

¼ cup mayonnaise
2 tablespoons
  yellow mustard
2 tablespoons allulose

This ketogenic take on a honey mustard sauce is sweet and savory but toned down with mayonnaise. The allulose closely mimics the flavor of honey, and its ability to easily dissolve in most liquids makes it the secret ingredient in this honey mustard clone.

In a small bowl, combine the mayonnaise, mustard, and allulose. Using a small whisk, mix the sauce until the allulose is completely dissolved, then use as desired.

Storage Tip: Any leftover sauce can be stored in an airtight container in the refrigerator for up to 1 week.

Macronutrients: 96% Fat, 2% Protein, 2% Carbs

Per serving (2 tablespoons): Calories: 98; Total Fat: 11g; Protein: 0g; Total Carbohydrates: 1g; Fiber: 0g; Erythritol: 0g; Allulose: 6g; Net Carbs: 1g

Greek Dressing

DAIRY FREE, EGG FREE, NUT FREE, UNDER 30 MINUTES, VEGETARIAN

Makes ½ cup
Prep Time: 2 minutes

¼ cup extra-virgin olive oil

2 tablespoons red
wine vinegar

1 garlic clove, minced

1 teaspoon freshly
squeezed lemon juice

1 teaspoon dried oregano

1 teaspoon dried parsley

½ teaspoon pink Himalayan
sea salt

¼ teaspoon freshly ground
black pepper

If you're looking for a simple yet flavorful vinaigrette, Greek dressing might just fit the bill. This dressing has a bright and fresh flavor, with plenty of fat for the keto diet. The herbs and spices infuse the dressing, making the perfect dressing for a simple salad.

In a small glass canning jar, combine the olive oil, vinegar, garlic, lemon juice, oregano, parsley, salt, and pepper. Shake well, then use as desired.

Storage Tip: Any leftover dressing can be stored in an airtight container in the refrigerator for up to 1 week.

Macronutrients: 98% Fat, 0% Protein, 2% Carbs

Per serving (2 tablespoons): Calories: 123; Total Fat: 14g; Protein: 0g; Total Carbohydrates: 1g; Fiber: 0g; Erythritol: 0g; Net Carbs: 1g

Hollandaise Sauce

NUT FREE, UNDER 30 MINUTES, VEGETARIAN

Makes about ¾ cup
Prep Time: 5 minutes
Cook Time: 5 minutes

½ cup (1 stick) butter
2 large egg yolks
1 tablespoon water
2 teaspoons freshly
 squeezed lemon juice
Pink Himalayan sea salt
Cayenne pepper
Ground white pepper

Hollandaise is a mixture of egg yolk, butter, and lemon juice. In other words, a fantastic sauce for the keto diet! It's simple to make and tastes amazing on eggs. The sauce feels creamy thanks to the egg yolk, but its flavor is what makes this special. You'll definitely taste the butter, but the lemon juice and cayenne are what make the sauce really pop.

1. In a medium saucepan, melt the butter over medium heat.

2. In a small bowl, combine the egg yolks, water, and lemon juice.

3. Reduce the heat to low under the saucepan, and slowly drizzle in the egg mixture while stirring. Continue to whisk the sauce over low heat until it thickens.

4. Season with the salt, cayenne, and white pepper.

Macronutrients: 96% Fat, 3% Protein, 1% Carbs

Per serving (3 tablespoons): Calories: 230; Total Fat: 25g; Protein: 2g; Total Carbohydrates: 1g; Fiber: 0g; Erythritol: 0g; Net Carbs: 1g

Beef Bone Broth

DAIRY FREE, EGG FREE, NUT FREE, ONE POT

Makes 6 cups
Prep Time: 5 minutes
Cook Time: 6 to 8 hours

2 pounds beef soup bones

6 cups water

¼ medium onion

1 celery stalk

1 tablespoon apple
cider vinegar

2 teaspoons black
peppercorns

1 teaspoon minced garlic

1 bay leaf

Pink Himalayan sea salt

Bone broth is a staple of the ketogenic diet. Not only do people cook with it, but many also drink it like tea. Often, it is recommended to keto beginners to help fight off the "keto flu." Whatever the reason, the broth has to be good enough to sip. This is rich in beef flavor, with hints of onion, celery, and garlic. You'll need a slow cooker for this recipe.

1. In a slow cooker, combine the bones, water, onion, celery, vinegar, peppercorns, garlic, bay leaf, and salt.

2. Cover and cook on the high setting for 6 to 8 hours. The longer you cook it, the more flavorful the broth will be.

3. Using a mesh strainer, strain the contents of the slow cooker into a large bowl. Discard the solids, and season the broth with salt.

Storage Tip: The broth can be stored in an airtight container in the refrigerator for up to 5 days.

Ingredient Tip: Soup bones are ideal for this recipe, but I often don't feel like paying for bones. My butcher is usually willing to give me bags of scrap bones for free. These turn into a great broth, but you might have to skim off a fat layer.

Macronutrients: 3% Fat, 96% Protein, 1% Carbs

Per serving (1½ cups): Calories: 60; Total Fat: 0g; Protein: 15g; Total Carbohydrates: 0g; Fiber: 0g; Erythritol: 0g; Net Carbs: 0g

Keto Bread

DAIRY FREE, VEGETARIAN

Serves 4
Prep Time: 5 minutes
Cook Time: 80 minutes

---

1 cup almond flour

⅓ cup coconut flour

¼ cup golden flax meal

2 tablespoons psyllium
husk powder

1 teaspoon cream of tartar

1 teaspoon baking soda

1 teaspoon active dry yeast
(optional)

½ teaspoon pink Himalayan
sea salt

1 cup warm water

3 large egg whites

1 large egg

1 tablespoon apple cider
vinegar or freshly
squeezed lemon juice

1 teaspoon extra-virgin
olive oil

Making a true keto bread is no easy undertaking. After about three months of trying, I finally perfected this recipe. The keto mini loaf is made without use of a bread pan or special tools. The texture is closer to rye bread than to white, and the slices are large enough to make a sandwich. Thanks to the addition of some yeast for flavor, you might actually forget you're eating keto bread.

1. Preheat the oven to 350°F. Line a baking sheet with parchment paper.

2. In a large bowl, combine the almond flour, coconut flour, flax meal, psyllium husk powder, cream of tartar, baking soda, yeast, and salt. Using a whisk, break up any clumps.

3. In a medium bowl, combine the water, egg whites, whole egg, vinegar, and olive oil. Whisk until the eggs are beaten and the liquid is smooth.

4. Pour the wet ingredients into the dry ingredients and quickly mix. The coconut flour will absorb a lot of liquid, and the baking soda will activate to create a stiff dough.

5. Transfer the dough to the baking sheet and form into a tall rectangular loaf. I like to form it into a "tombstone" shape so that the slices are large enough for a sandwich; it will bake, but it won't rise, as would a yeast-risen wheat bread.

CONTINUES ▶

6. Bake for 75 to 80 minutes, then let cool for 1 hour. Slice as desired.

Storage Tip: Any leftover bread will keep in a resealable plastic bag in the refrigerator for up to 1 week. The bread can be frozen to keep even longer.

Macronutrients: 61% Fat, 19% Protein, 20% Carbs

Per serving: Calories: 279; Total Fat: 19g; Protein: 13g; Total Carbohydrates: 14g; Fiber: 8g; Erythritol: 0g; Net Carbs: 6g

Cheesy Garlic Biscuits

UNDER 30 MINUTES, VEGETARIAN

Makes 2 biscuits
Prep Time: 5 minutes
Cook Time: 12 minutes

For the biscuits

¼ cup almond flour

¼ cup grated
    cheddar cheese

1 teaspoon baking powder

¼ teaspoon pink Himalayan
    sea salt

¼ teaspoon garlic powder

1 large egg

2 tablespoons
    butter, melted

1 tablespoon heavy
    (whipping) cream

For the topping

1 tablespoon butter, melted

¼ teaspoon dried parsley

Pinch of garlic powder

If you're missing biscuits on your keto diet, here is the solution. These are stable enough to hold together but still have that nice crumble we expect from a biscuit. They're infused with the rich flavors of garlic, cheddar, and butter before being baked to a beautiful golden-brown color.

1. Preheat the oven to 425°F. Line a baking sheet with parchment paper.

2. **To make the biscuits:** In a medium bowl, combine the almond flour, cheese, baking powder, salt, and garlic powder.

3. In a small bowl, combine the egg, butter, and cream. Whisk the mixture until the egg is beaten.

4. Pour the wet ingredients into the dry, then mix just enough to combine the ingredients to form a dough.

5. Divide the dough in half and place both pieces on the baking sheet with a little space between.

6. Bake for 10 to 12 minutes, until the biscuits are golden brown tipped with a darker brown.

7. **To make the topping:** In a small bowl, combine the butter, parsley, and garlic powder. Brush the biscuits with the butter mixture, then serve immediately.

> **Variation Tip:** The spices and cheese can be swapped out for any others you can imagine. You can even add a bit of diced jalapeño to create a spicy cheese biscuit.

Macronutrients: 84% Fat, 11% Protein, 5% Carbs

Per serving (1 biscuit): Calories: 344; Total Fat: 33g; Protein: 9g; Total Carbohydrates: 5g; Fiber: 2g; Erythritol: 0g; Net Carbs: 3g

Keto Tortillas

DAIRY FREE, EGG FREE, UNDER 30 MINUTES, VEGETARIAN

Makes 4 tortillas
Prep Time: 10 minutes
Cook Time: 10 minutes

⅔ cup water

½ cup coconut flour

⅓ cup golden flax meal

3 tablespoons extra-virgin olive oil

1½ teaspoons xanthan gum

¼ teaspoon pink Himalayan sea salt

There is nothing wrong with buying keto tortillas, but they can be hard to find in some places. Thanks to my love for anything wrapped in a tortilla, I was able to devise this recipe. The finished tortilla holds together incredibly well and has a mouthfeel similar to a flour tortilla. It will go well with whatever you choose to fill it with.

1. In a medium bowl, combine the water, coconut flour, flax meal, olive oil, xanthan gum, and salt.

2. Divide the dough into 4 equal portions.

3. Place each dough ball between 2 sheets of parchment paper, then roll the dough into a $\frac{1}{16}$- to $\frac{1}{8}$-inch-thick round.

4. Heat a griddle pan over medium heat. Place each tortilla on the griddle pan and cook for 60 seconds on each side, then transfer the tortilla to a plate. Cover the tortillas with a towel to retain the moisture.

5. Serve immediately or let cool for use later.

Storage Tip: Store these tortillas in a resealable 1-gallon plastic bag in the refrigerator for up to 1 week.

Macronutrients: 68% Fat, 9% Protein, 23% Carbs

Per serving (1 tortilla): Calories: 212; Total Fat: 16g; Protein: 5g; Total Carbohydrates: 12g; Fiber: 7g; Erythritol: 0g; Net Carbs: 5g

Measurement Conversions

	US Standard	US Standard (ounces)	Metric (approximate)
Volume Equivalents (Liquid)	2 tablespoons	1 fl. oz.	30 mL
	¼ cup	2 fl. oz.	60 mL
	½ cup	4 fl. oz.	120 mL
	1 cup	8 fl. oz.	240 mL
	1½ cups	12 fl. oz.	355 mL
	2 cups or 1 pint	16 fl. oz.	475 mL
	4 cups or 1 quart	32 fl. oz.	1 L
	1 gallon	128 fl. oz.	4 L
Volume Equivalents (Dry)	⅛ teaspoon		0.5 mL
	¼ teaspoon		1 mL
	½ teaspoon		2 mL
	¾ teaspoon		4 mL
	1 teaspoon		5 mL
	1 tablespoon		15 mL
	¼ cup		59 mL
	⅓ cup		79 mL
	½ cup		118 mL
	⅔ cup		156 mL
	¾ cup		177 mL
	1 cup		235 mL
	2 cups or 1 pint		475 mL
	3 cups		700 mL
	4 cups or 1 quart		1 L
	½ gallon		2 L
	1 gallon		4 L
Weight Equivalents	½ ounce		15 g
	1 ounce		30 g
	2 ounces		60 g
	4 ounces		115 g
	8 ounces		225 g
	12 ounces		340 g
	16 ounces or 1 pound		455 g

	Fahrenheit (F)	Celsius (C) (Approximate)
Oven Temperatures	250°F	120°F
	300°F	150°C
	325°F	180°C
	375°F	190°C
	400°F	200°C
	425°F	220°C
	450°F	230°C

Resources

WEBSITES

Black Sheep Keto: For additional information on the keto diet, and more recipes, visit BlackSheepKeto.com.

KetoCon: While I could name a million resources on the keto diet, KetoCon gathers them all under one roof. If you're interested in the science of keto, this is a good place to start.

KETO BRANDS

Kite Hill: Kite Hills makes an almond yogurt that can be used for several of the recipes in this book. The plain flavor is keto friendly, but be sure to check the nutrition label on any of the fruit flavors.

Lakanto: Lakanto makes one of my favorite sweeteners for keto. It is a blend of monkfruit and erythritol that tastes much closer to sugar than plain erythritol. Plus, it will convert 1:1 in any recipe in this book. They also make a powdered variety.

Lily's: When it comes to chocolate chips and chocolate bars, I have not found anything that tastes better or is more easily available than Lily's. Sweetened with stevia and erythritol, their chocolates are perfect for the keto diet.

Miracle Noodle: Whether you call them shirataki or konjac noodles, they're almost synonymous with the brand Miracle Noodle. As one of the original manufacturers of shirataki noodles, Miracle Noodle makes a great product. I keep a few of these on hand for all my pasta needs.

Two Good: Two Good yogurt is the best keto yogurt. I prefer this in my smoothies and parfaits. Thanks to the popularity of low-carb diets, I can find this at my local store.

Walden Farms: Walden Farms makes a wide variety of keto sauces. While some of them are hit or miss, their pancake syrup is amazing. When a recipe calls for maple-flavored syrup, this is it.

References

Allulose Sweetener. Allulose.org.

D'Andrea Meira, I., Romão, T. T., Pires do Prado, H. J., Krüger, L. T., Pires, M., and da Conceição, P. O. "Ketogenic Diet and Epilepsy: What We Know So Far." *Frontiers in Neuroscience* 13, no. 5 (2019). https://doi.org/10.3389/fnins.2019.00005.

Davis, D. R., Epp, M. D., and Riordan, H. D. "Changes in USDA Food Composition Data for 43 Garden Crops, 1950 to 1999." *Journal of the American College of Nutrition* 23, no. 6 (December 2004): 669–82. doi: 10.1080/07315724.2004.10719409

D'Andrea Meira, I., Romão, T. T., Pires do Prado, H. J., Krüger, L. T., Pires, M., & da Conceição, P. O. (2019). Ketogenic Diet and Epilepsy: What We Know So Far. *Frontiers in neuroscience*, 13, 5. https://doi.org/10.3389/fnins.2019.00005

Rauchhaus, M., Clark, A. L., Doehner, W., Davos, C., Bolger, A., Sharma, R., and Anker, S. D. "The Relationship Between Cholesterol and Survival in Patients with Chronic Heart Failure." *Journal of the American College of Cardiology* 42, no. 11 (December 3, 2003): 1933–40. doi: 10.1016/j.jacc.2003.07.016

Yancy, W. S., Jr., Foy, M., Chalecki, A. M., Vernon, M. C., and Westman, E. C. "A Low-Carbohydrate, Ketogenic Diet to Treat Type 2 Diabetes." *Nutrition and Metabolism* 2, no. 34 (2205). doi.org/10.1186/1743-7075-2-34.

Index

Acknowledgments

When I started writing this book, I had no idea how much work I was in for. This challenge was elevated further by the COVID-19 pandemic, which left many ingredients and services hard to come by. For this reason, I owe a lot of credit to my wife, Olivia, and my long-time friend Robert. Without Olivia's help I would have had far fewer ingredients in my fridge and a mountain of dishes in the sink. Her dedication to tracking down hard-to-find ingredients truly made this book possible.

Robert has contributed greatly to my success as both a social-media influencer and author of this book. As one of the first people I ever coached on keto, he has taught me a lot about how to make this diet work for anyone who has the drive to follow it. In true Robert fashion, he came through with my author photograph for this book when no one else would.

Finally, I would like to thank the entire team at Callisto Media for all their hard work on this project. It has been amazing to see my words and recipes transformed into such a clean and polished book. Without their expertise and guidance, the book in your hand would never have been written.

About the Author

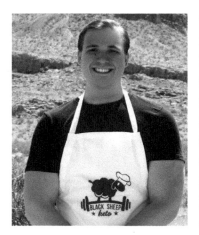

Thomas Martens is the creative mind behind Black Sheep Keto and BlackSheepKeto.com, where he produces recipes and shares information about the ketogenic diet. Tom has influenced tens of thousands of people to start the keto diet through his social-media following. Though he is not formally trained as a chef, Tom's recipes have quickly gained popularity online, and many hold front-page search results on YouTube. As a true keto success story, his passion for the ketogenic diet and recipe creation began in 2015, when he started the ketogenic diet in an attempt to control his ever-increasing waistline. Five years, one hundred pounds, and hundreds of hours of recipe experimentation later, Tom wrote the *Ketogenic Diet for Two* cookbook as a way to spread his recipes to a wider audience and, ultimately, help more people achieve their weight-loss goals.

CPSIA information can be obtained
at www.ICGtesting.com
Printed in the USA
JSHW030049090820
7153JS00010B/14